Medical Technology into Healthcare and Society

Health, Technology and Society

Series Editors: **Andrew Webster**, University of York, UK and **Sally Wyatt**, Royal Netherlands Academy of Arts and Sciences, The Netherlands

Titles include:

Gerard de Vries and Klasien Horstman (*editors*)
GENETICS FROM LABORATORY TO SOCIETY
Societal Learning as an Alternative to Regulation

Alex Faulkner
MEDICAL TECHNOLOGY INTO HEALTHCARE AND SOCIETY
A Sociology of Devices, Innovation and Governance

Jessica Mesman
MEDICAL INNOVATION AND UNCERTAINTY IN NEONATOLOGY

Nadine Wathen, Sally Wyatt and Roma Harris (*editors*)
MEDIATING HEALTH INFORMATION
The Go-Betweens in a Changing Socio-Technical Landscape

Andrew Webster (*editor*)
NEW TECHNOLOGIES IN HEALTH CARE
Challenge, Change and Innovation

Forthcoming titles include:

John Abraham and Courtney Davis
CHALLENGING PHARMACEUTICAL REGULATION
Innovation and Public Health in Europe and the United States

Herbert Gottweis, Brian Salter and Catherine Waldby
THE GLOBAL POLITICS OF HUMAN EMBRYONIC STEM CELL SCIENCE

Maggie Mort, Tracy Finch, Carl May and Frances Mair
MOBILISING MEDICINE
Information Technology and the Modernisation of Health Care

Steven P. Wainwright and Clare Williams
THE BODY, BIO-MEDICINE AND SOCIETY
Reflections on High-Tech Medicine

Health, Technology and Society
Series Standing Order ISBN 978-1–4039–9131–7 hardback
(*outside North America only*)

You can receive future titles in this series as they are published by placing a standing order. Please contact your bookseller or, in case of difficulty, write to us at the address below with your name and address, the title of the series and the ISBN quoted above.

Customer Services Department, Macmillan Distribution Ltd, Houndmills, Basingstoke, Hampshire RG21 6XS, England

---

Medical Technology into Healthcare and Society

A Sociology of Devices, Innovation and Governance

Alex Faulkner
Cardiff University, UK

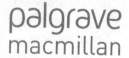

First published 2009 by
PALGRAVE MACMILLAN

Palgrave Macmillan in the UK is an imprint of Macmillan Publishers Limited,
registered in England, company number 785998, of Houndmills, Basingstoke,
Hampshire RG21 6XS.

Palgrave Macmillan in the US is a division of St Martin's Press LLC,
175 Fifth Avenue, New York, NY 10010.

Palgrave Macmillan is the global academic imprint of the above companies
and has companies and representatives throughout the world.

Palgrave® and Macmillan® are registered trademarks in the United States,
the United Kingdom, Europe and other countries.

ISBN-13: 978-0-230-00171-8   hardback
ISBN-10: 0-230-00171-8   hardback

This book is printed on paper suitable for recycling and made from fully
managed and sustained forest sources. Logging, pulping and manufacturing
processes are expected to conform to the environmental regulations of the
country of origin.

A catalogue record for this book is available from the British Library.

Library of Congress Cataloging-in-Publication Data

Faulkner, Alex, 1952–
  Medical technology into healthcare and society: a sociology of devices,
    innovation and governance / Alex Faulkner.
      p. ; cm.—(Health, technology, and society)
  Includes bibliographical references and index.
  ISBN-13: 978-0-230-00171-8 (hardback : alk. paper)
  ISBN-10: 0-230-00171-8 (hardback : alk. paper)   1. Medical
  instruments and apparatus—Social aspects.   2. Medical
innovations—Social aspects.   I. Title.   II. Series.
  [DNLM: 1. Equipment and Supplies—standards.   2. Health Policy.
  3. Technology, Medical—standards. W 26 F263m 2008]
  R856.F38 2008
  610.28–dc22   2008024581

10   9   8   7   6   5   4   3   2   1
18   17   16   15   14   13   12   11   10   09

Printed and bound in Great Britain by
CPI Antony Rowe, Chippenham and Eastbourne

*In memory of my father, who liked conundrums,
and of my mother, who saw no point in them*

Contents

Figures

Tables

ix

Preface

Medical devices are the Cinderella of technologies in the healthcare sector. The world of medical devices has a low profile in the public sphere compared to pharmaceuticals. While medical *technology* receives increasing attention, the significance of *devices* as a sector in healthcare systems and in wider society remains a relatively neglected topic in social science analysis and interpretation.

In the context of this relative neglect, this book has several aims. First, it aims to shed light on the relatively invisible processes of production, promotion, adoption, governance and modification of medical device technologies. Second, it aims to conceptualise and illustrate the relationship between the 'evidence-based' movements that have become characteristic of public services in the advanced industrialised societies over the last 20 years and to contribute to understanding this movement in relation to the dynamics of healthcare governance between contemporary medical device industries, healthcare systems and society. Third, the book draws upon theory in sociology of technology, science and technology studies and regulatory governance, as well as the methods and approaches of the healthcare sciences themselves, with the aim of making some contributions to conceptual development in these fields.

My method is to draw on detailed comparative case studies of five devices that represent a range of configurations of device technology–healthcare system-evidence-regulation-users (and non-users). The case studies focus primarily on the UK and Europe, the European Union context being especially important for medical device regulation. The innovation and diffusion of these technologies all have elements of more or less controversy associated with them, although this was not my reason for selecting them.

Medical device technologies raise questions of risk and benefit both to health and to the healthcare system and its stakeholders. The social relations of governance of safety, efficacy/effectiveness and societal acceptability differ between the device technologies in ways that the book will illuminate. Innovation in biomaterials raises a number of questions about evidence for performance of material technology, the clinical and social practices in which they are deployed, the ways in which they may or may not enter the healthcare system, questions of advocacy and promotion between industry and policymakers and regulators and questions of clinical 'need' or utility.

The book does not set out directly to assess or suggest strategies for producing and diffusing device technologies that are *desirable* for health-care and society. This ambition has been very usefully tackled recently by Pascale Lehoux in *The Problem of Health Technology* (Lehoux, 2006) – especially the concluding chapter 'Toward Better Innovations', and to some extent by Andrew Webster's *Health Technology and Society: a socio-logical critique* (2007) and analysis of health technology assessment (Webster, 2004). A similar critique, emphasising the lack of attention to 'context' and an inability of technology assessment methods to assess the effectiveness on patient care of regulatory regimes, has come from the major political science analyst of the medical device sector in Europe (Altenstetter, 1996, 2004). I take it that these critiques should be taken seriously, and aim in my case study analyses to show the varying 'contexts' of different device technologies, in which societal desirability is negotiated between different stakeholder constituencies of healthcare systems and society.

I do not analyse the micro-politics of innovation of devices into the healthcare system at 'local' level, for example through the work of ethics committees, clinical championing and clinical trials, hospital-level con-tracting and purchasing, local clinical effectiveness evaluation and so on. Rather, the focus is on the broader processes of regulatory governance and stakeholder interactions that shape and are shaped by the differing innovation profiles of the particular devices on which I focus.

I hope the book will have appeal for several different audiences. Since the medical device sector and its modes of regulation are not well known, even in many parts of the healthcare system and the healthcare professions themselves, I hope that practitioners and policymakers in these fields will find it informative. For those clinical professionals with an interest in the fields of clinical practice represented by the case studies that I examine, I hope that the broad-ranging analysis of differ-ent dimensions of innovation, governance and what I call the 'usership' of the technology will be of interest. Each of the case study chapters ends with a short section discussing the dynamics of innovation, policy and governance in the field, and this is followed in each case by a sec-tion in which 'technology and society' issues are discussed from a more sociological perspective. I hope that this approach will make a contri-bution of value for policymakers and scholars in sociology and science and technology studies. I believe that the book as a whole offers a study in a particular politico-economic sector in which industrial economy meets public services, and that as such the analysis will be of value to those with an interest in technological innovation in cross-sectoral and cross-industry comparisons.

The structure of the book is as follows. In the first chapter, I introduce approaches and concepts that are useful for understanding the processes of innovation and governance that are to be found in science and technology and the contemporary 'regulatory state'. Here, I pay particular attention to the rise of what I call 'evidentiality' in the sphere of healthcare systems in the United Kingdom. In the following chapter, I critically introduce some key approaches and concepts from sociology and science and technology studies (STS) that I draw upon throughout the book. In the third chapter, I introduce 'the world of medical devices', giving attention to various aspects of the industrial sector and, especially, medical device regulation. This is followed by five case study chapters, four devoted to a very specific type of device technology, and the fifth discussing the boundary between what might be termed 'deviceness' and emerging bio-technology, by looking at the development of a regulatory regime for tissue engineering, one of the strands of the emerging paradigm of regenerative medicine. The final chapter then offers a comparative analysis of the case studies and discusses their significance in terms of concepts of society/technology studies: innovation pathways, governance, the 'usership' of technologies and forms of medicalisation in the evolving relationships between technology, healthcare and society.

Alex Faulkner, Cardiff

Series Preface

Medicine, healthcare and the wider social meaning and management of health are undergoing major changes. In part this reflects developments in science and technology, which enable new forms of diagnosis, treatment and the delivery of healthcare. It also reflects changes in the locus of care and burden of responsibility for health. Today, genetics, informatics, imaging and integrative technologies, such as nanotechnology, are redefining our understanding of the body, health and disease; at the same time, health is no longer simply the domain of conventional medicine, nor the clinic.

More broadly, the social management of health itself is losing its anchorage in collective social relations and shared knowledge and practice, whether at the level of the local community or through state-funded socialised medicine. This individualisation of health is both culturally driven and state sponsored, as the promotion of 'self-care' demonstrates. The very technologies that redefine health are also the means through which this individualisation can occur – through 'e-health', diagnostic tests and the commodification of restorative tissue, such as stem cells and cloned embryos.

This series explores these processes within and beyond the conventional domain of 'the clinic', and asks whether they amount to a qualitative shift in the social ordering and value of medicine and health. Locating technical developments in wider socio-economic and political processes, each text discusses and critiques recent developments within health technologies in specific areas, drawing on a range of analyses provided by the social sciences. Some will have a more theoretical, others a more applied focus, interrogating and contributing towards a health policy. All will draw on recent research conducted by the author(s).

The Health, Technology and Society Series also looks towards the medium term in anticipating the likely configurations of health in advanced industrial societies and does so comparatively, through exploring the globalisation and the internationalisation of health, health inequalities and their expression through existing and new social divisions.

This book makes a valuable contribution to the series in three ways. First, Faulkner offers rich empirical material about 'mundane' technologies that are used in everyday clinical practice, including artificial hips, the PSA test for prostate cancer, infusion pumps and coagulometers, as well as tissue engineering, a possible future mundane technology. Such everyday technologies receive relatively little scholarly and policy attention despite their enormous use in healthcare settings around the world. Second, on a theoretical level, Faulkner offers a timely and useful corrective to over-simple analyses of the co-construction of society and technology by illustrating how this process may be uneven and how it differs considerably across distinct socio-material domains within the medical devices arena. Third, the book includes a policy-related strand that offers a critique of healthcare science/HTA (health technology assessment) and its role in evaluating the utility of these different technologies. The richness of the case studies reveals how patchy, provisional and uncertain these evaluations and the technologies actually are.

Andrew Webster and Sally Wyatt

Acknowledgements

This book owes its intellectual and empirical origins to two main sources. First, I worked in the areas of health technology assessment and health services research during the 1990s at the Department of Social Medicine, University of Bristol, UK, and I am grateful for the range of insight into different health technologies which I gained there. My interest in artificial hips and prostate cancer testing stems from that period. Second, during my time at the Cardiff School of Social Sciences, Cardiff University, Wales, UK, I have been grateful for the opportunity to engage with a stimulating environment including scholars in the social studies of science and technology and medical sociology. I particularly thank Mick Bloor for his support. I am grateful for the support provided by the Cardiff School in providing time which I could devote to this book. Some of the analytic ideas in the book were formed as part of my PhD by Published Work at Edinburgh University, and I thank Sarah Cunningham-Burley for her advice there. My interest in medical device regulation as a sociological topic has benefited particularly from collaborative working and writing with Julie Kent, of the University of the West of England. Clinical engineer–public health researcher Mara Souza worked with me for a year as part of her sandwich PhD based in Salvador, Brazil – I thank her for her energy, enthusiasm and major contribution to Chapter 6.

I thank a number of people and organisations for permission to use material quoted or reproduced in the book. In particular, I am grateful to Jenny Donovan of the Department of Social Medicine, Bristol, for permission to quote from her unpublished study of orthopaedic surgeons' and hip prostheses, and for research conversations about Health Technology Assessment of prostate cancer testing and treatment. Chris Gardiner of the Department of Health's Device Evaluation Centre kindly provided detailed information and views about his area of work. I am grateful for the opportunity to access the growing archival materials of the Centre for History of Evaluation in Health Care (CHEHC) held at Cardiff University library, where I looked at the papers of Professor Sir Miles Irving relating to his time as the first chair of the UK's Standing Group on Health Technology.

Chapter 8 of the book is based largely on research conducted with the support of the UK's Economic and Social Research Council

(ESRC) Innovative Health Technologies programme, award number L218252058, and non-programme grant RES-000-22-1814. Here I also thank my research team colleagues, Julie Kent, Ingrid Geesink, David FitzPatrick and Peter Glasner.

For permission to reproduce graphic materials, I thank Eve Knight of Anticoagulation Europe; Wellcome Images; the NHS Centre for Reviews and Dissemination; Dr Lindsay Grant of Royal United Hospital, Bath; the National Audit Office; (Organogenesis)

The book would have been impossible without the support, curiosity, tolerance and humour of my family as I sat down with the 'pages' or 'chapter' (the word 'book' was banned because it implied an excessive task). My thanks and appreciation here go especially to Margaret, and to my daughters Martha and Ruth.

Abbreviations

ABHI	Association of British Healthcare Industries
ACE	Anticoagulation Europe
ACI	Articular Cartilage Implantation
AF	Atrial Fibrillation
ANT	Actor-Network Theory
ANVISA	National Health Surveillance Agency (Brazil)
BAUS	British Association of Urological Surgeons
BHS	British Hip Society
BIME	Bath Institute of Medical Engineering
BOA	British Orthopaedic Association
BPH	Benign Prostatic Hypertrophy
BSI	British Standards Institute
BUPA	British United Provident Association
CEN	European Committee for Standardisation
CEP	Centre for Evidence-based Purchasing (part of NHS PASA)
CHeF	CEN Healthcare Forum
CHEHC	Centre for the History of Evaluation in Health Care (Cardiff University)
CSD	Committee for the Safety of Devices (MHRA)
DEC	Device Evaluation Centre
DES	Device Evaluation Service
DRE	Digital Rectal Examination
DVT	Deep Vein Thrombosis
EBM	Evidence-Based Medicine
EC	European Commission
ECRI	ECRI Institute: US non-profit HTA organisation
EMEA	European Medicines Agency
ENVI	Committee of the Environment, Public Health and Consumer Protection (European Parliament)
EU	European Union
EUCOMED	European Confederation of Medical Device Associations
FDA	Food and Drug Administration (US)
FMEA	Failure Mode Effect Analysis
GP	General medical practitioner

GCP	Good Clinical Practice
GMP	Good Manufacturing Practice
HITF	Healthcare Industries Task Force
HSR	Health Services Research
HTA	Health Technology Assessment
HTEP	Human Tissue Engineered Product
ICT	Information and Communication Technology
IEC	International Electrotechnical Commission
INR	International Normalized Ratio
IPTS	Institute for Prospective Technological Studies (see JRS)
ISO	International Standards Organization
IV	Intravenous
IVMDD	In Vitro Medical Device Directive
JRC	Joint Research Centre (of European Commission)
LUTS	Lower Urinary Tract Syndrome
MDA	Medical Device Agency (now MHRA)
MDD	Medical Device Directive
MHRA	Medicines and Healthcare products Regulatory Agency, UK
MRC	Medical Research Council
NAO	National Audit Office
NHS	National Health Service
NHS Trust	UK NHS healthcare provider
NHSCRD	NHS Centre for Reviews and Dissemination
NICE	National Institute for Health and Clinical Excellence
NJR	National Joint Registry
NPSA	National Patient Safety Agency
NSC	National Screening Commitee
OAT	Oral Anticoagulation
ODEP	Orthopaedic Data Evaluation Panel (NHS PASA)
PASA	(NHS) Purchasing and Supply Agency
PCRMP	Prostate Cancer Risk Management Programme
PCT	Primary Care Trust (UK, NHS)
POCT	Point-of-care Testing
PROM	Patient Reported Outcome Measurement
PSA	Prostate-Specific Antigen
PSM	Patient Self-Monitoring
PTCA	Percutaneous Transluminary Coronary Angioplasty
RCN	Royal College of Nursing
RCS	Royal College of Surgeons
RCT	Randomised Control Trial

SCOT	Social Construction of Technology
SCMPMD	Scientific Committee on Medicinal Products and Medical Devices (European Commission)
SIMPATIE	Safety Improvement for Patients In Europe (project)
SME	Small and Medium-sized Enterprise
STS	Science and Technology Studies
TE	Tissue Engineering
THR	Total Hip Replacement
UKXIRA	United Kingdom Xenotransplantation Interim Authority
VTBI	Volume To Be Administered (infusion)
WHO	World Health Organization

1

Innovation, Evidence and Governance of Medical Technology

Introduction

Contemporary healthcare is characterised by what the UK government in the 1990s saw as a 'tidal wave' of innovation in health technology. Healthcare sciences and regulatory institutions for steering innovation have, over the last 20 years, been a notable social and political accompaniment to this tidal wave. Medical technologies are the product of global industries and the object of multidimensional promotion and regulation. Contemporary technological healthcare is characterised by a multitude of medical devices, ranging from the bandage to the bioreactor, the thermometer to magnetic resonance imaging, from the cancer-screening test to the heart pacemaker and to human cell and tissue therapies. These technologies are hugely different from each other as artefacts, but the ways in which they are promoted and controlled in societies and economies have notable consistencies.

Many, though not all, of the ubiquitous technologies of healthcare are medical devices. The terminology of 'devices' invokes attention to the institutionalised medical device industries and sectors, and medical device regulation and governance processes. Innovation of medical device technologies into the healthcare system is a process in which a variety of social, economic and medical interests and visions meet. The pursuit of medical innovation interests is typically conflictual, and often controversial. The 'evidence-based' movements in public policy and practice have grown over the last 20 years – methodologically and institutionally – nowhere more than in healthcare. At the same time, governments and healthcare policymakers espouse a doctrine of modernisation that promotes continual innovation in medical technology and practice. Innovation holds the potential to engender improved quality and effectiveness of healthcare services, but as May et al. (2001) have pointed out, this commitment to modernisation in contemporary healthcare policy often comes into conflict with the commitment to an evidence base for policy decisions. Indeed, it is paradoxical that a high level of innovation in healthcare provision is central to the growth of the new healthcare sciences during the 1990s, which brings a radical science-based questioning of the evidential basis on which innovation decisions are made, following rationalist experimental knowledge methodologies (Faulkner, 1997; Harrison, 1998). An analysis of healthcare innovation that conceptualises the dynamics of state and stakeholder actions to regulate and control innovation in the healthcare system must, therefore, accord the new healthcare sciences themselves a prime position. The agendas and knowledge products of the healthcare sciences have become closely tied to healthcare policymaking in a form of 'regulatory science' (Irwin et al., 1997). Evidence-based healthcare should thus be conceptualised as a phenomenon of political regulation and social legitimation as well as a scientific movement.

Health hazards and the societal apprehension of 'risk' have assumed an extraordinarily large place in the analysis of contemporary healthcare systems and public health (e.g. Lupton, 1995; Petersen, 1996; Howson, 1998; Robertson, 2000) and of course in social theory more broadly, for example in Beck's (1992) hypothesis of the risk society. The case studies discussed in this book have a concern with hazards and the production of risks associated with healthcare itself, in medical terminology sometimes called iatrogenic risk, and given its most extreme formulation in the early work of Illich (1975), a viewpoint that remains highly relevant to contemporary healthcare (Edwards, 1999). As will be demonstrated, the assessment of risks of technical performance, safety and efficacy of medical devices is a key part of the evolving regimes of evidence-related governance. This will be shown in, for example, case studies of hip prostheses, the PSA (prostate-specific antigen) test for prostate cancer and infusion pumps. Risk assessment has become increasingly important to an understanding of contemporary medical technology governance processes. It has been suggested that Europe faces a general shift towards more risk-averse and more stringent regulatory policies (Vogel, 2001) enshrined in policy movements such as the precautionary principle. However, there is some evidence of counter-trends, for example in pharmaceuticals regulation (Abraham and Davis, 2007), suggesting that the development of regulatory regimes and judgements of whether they are becoming more or less stringent should be subject to empirical analysis of specific sectors, technologies and devices.

In this chapter, I briefly review some of the key contributions to the study of technological innovation that are useful to approaching medical device technology, and I note the recent formulations of 'governance' and the 'regulatory state' that indicate important shifts in the forms of government associated with the massively varying forms of contemporary technological healthcare.

Innovation systems and pathways

Innovation processes have been conceptualised in many different ways by different academic disciplines. In this section, I briefly present some of the concepts that have been used to understand technology innovation processes and 'innovation systems', with special reference to medical technology. Some of this work overlaps with the sociological approaches discussed in Chapter 2 below. The perception that innovation occurs in 'systems' that display particular forms of organisation, resourcing, expertise, interinstitutional relationships and so on, is important to a consideration of medical devices, because innovation in the medical device industry – sectors or technological 'zones' – can be characterised as quite distinctive, and very different from other industrial sectors producing health technologies, notably pharmaceuticals (van Merode et al., 2002).

Processes of innovation of technologies into healthcare display some broad structural features. For example, it is established that the rate of adoption of new medical technology into the British healthcare system during the last decades of the twentieth century was slower and narrower than that of, for example, Germany and the US (Moran, 1999). As Moran noted, this was not due to a rational and effective gatekeeping function performed on the basis of scientifically based technology assessment. Rather, the relatively slow adoption was associated with the structuring effects of fixed budgets in the public system and the 'command and control', bureaucratic, monolithic form of healthcare delivery and strategy making, that was dismantled by the marketising reforms as the 1990s progressed.

Technological innovation in an industrial economy contends with conflicting forces of sectoralisation and 'networks' of innovation. National and supranational states orient themselves towards trading sectors and their representatives in negotiating industrial innovation policy and resourcing. Such sectoral organisation may cross-cut what is increasingly conceived as the 'distributed' nature of technological innovation, which has been well evidenced in some fields of medical device development (cf. Ramlogan et al., 2007). The development of novel forms of innovation networks in science and technology in the advanced capitalist societies has been noted in concepts of 'strategic alliance' between university research and healthcare companies (Webster, 1994) and the 'triple helix' of industry, academia and state (Etzkowitz and Leydesdorff, 2002). Distributed or interactive innovation processes have been depicted as 'depending crucially on the ability to integrate knowledge through networks linking distributed arrays of specialist groups, professions and organisations', and 'on the institutional context in which they unfold' (Swan et al., 2007). This characterisation has much in common with the concept of the 'technological zone' that I discuss at the end of Chapter 2, and which informs much of the discussion in this book. The boundaries of sectors may intersect with those of technological zones, and should not be conceived as fixed and immutable. Indeed, it is one of the recurring themes of the case studies of medical devices in this book that the social and material boundary-definitions of technologies are constantly being redefined through society's role in innovation of biomaterials, and combination and convergence between disparate technologies.

Understanding of sectoral systems of innovation and production has been developed especially from an evolutionary economics perspective (Malerba, 2004, 2006). Malerba (1999) has outlined a range of 'heterogeneous actors' involved in the evolution of an innovating sector: 'Firms, universities, government agencies, research institutes, industrial association, entrepreneurs, consumers, financial institutions, trade unions'. As Malerba notes, however, the sectoral systems approach 'places emphasis on the role of non-firm organizations such as universities, financial institutions, government, local authorities and of institutions and rules of the games such as standards, regulations, labor markets and so on'. These differ greatly in their configuration across sectors. More recently, the *emergence* of new sectoral systems has been identified as a key area for further research (Malerba, 2006). Although referring to government agencies, this approach does not accord regulatory policymaking and regime-building the constructive, shaping status that they deserve. This concern will be a constant focus throughout this book, and I will argue that regulatory regime-building has a constructive effect – establishing 'rules of the game' through standards and other organising principles – as well as a blueprinting effect in shaping the innovation pathways of medical technologies (cf. Bud, 1999; Faulkner, forthcoming). A similar approach to the dynamic role of the institutions of state – as well as by greater incorporation of notions of the usership of technology – has also been recommended in a conceptual model that brings together sociology and institutional analysis (Geels, 2005). This strand of analysis will be particularly highlighted in the chapter discussing 'regulatory innovation' in the technological zone of tissue engineering (Faulkner et al., 2006).

Convergence between technologies is of growing importance. A notable contribution to the research literature on the 'shapers' of technology has been the concept of 'technological system' first elaborated by historian Hughes (1983), and subsequently taken up widely in science and technology studies. Interdependence between technologies is highlighted in this approach, which emphasises the interweaving of the social and the technical into patterned systems in the pathways of technology innovation. Hughes's work has been presented in relation to the 'social shaping' approaches as representing 'the technological shaping of technology' (MacKenzie and Wajcman, 1999). This and related approaches to understanding technology in society are discussed further in Chapter 2.

Innovation pathways

An early study of the social control of technology (Collingridge, 1980) discussed the dilemma of how technologies are typically relatively 'fluid' in their early phases when they might be altered comparatively easily, but their social implications at this point are relatively difficult to discern. At later stages, they become more rigid but by that point their social implications, although possibly better known, become less amenable to intervention. This analysis was an early example of concepts of 'lock-in' and 'path-dependence', which are now important to any analysis of the pathways that technology innovation might take. These concepts acknowledge the salience of the resilience ('obduracy') of the pathway taken by established technological systems. When considering innovation pathways and potentially emerging technologies, sectors or technological zones, these concepts of directionality have been developed in the notion of emerging 'irreversibilities' (van Merkerk and van Lente, 2005). In this approach, concepts of socio-technological 'expectations' and agenda-setting are key to the early-emerging phase of new technologies. Irreversibilities may be found at three interrelated levels: the basic research group or firm, the scientific–technological field and society (van Merkerk and van Lente, 2005: 1108); this book focuses on the latter two levels. Also emphasised in this approach is the importance of networks of actors in early innovation processes (van Merkerk and Robinson, 2006).

Thus the idea of multifaceted, directional, interlocking social and technological processes is key to an understanding of the developmental pathway that particular medical devices might take in entering and becoming adopted in healthcare settings.

Similar attempts to understand the relationships between product design and society are seen in novel developments of 'activity theory' that have emerged especially in academic work coming from Scandinavia. This considers the relation between collective product design processes and the resulting artefacts. For example, Hyysalo has usefully attempted to improve on the important concept of the directive 'technological frame' that was elaborated by Bijker (1995).[1] He proposes the notion of 'practice-bound imaginary' to refer to ways in which innovatory design practices are both motivated and restricted by practices that 'bundle collective expectations' which 'create a sense of direction' in technological design projects (Hyysalo, 2004, 2006). This approach valuably focuses on the interacting groups and organisations involved in design, highlighting *producer–user* relations in the development of devices, and challenging taken-for-granted notions of clear boundaries between designers/developers and users (Hyysalo, op. cit.). I take up this point again in the 'co-constructionist' contributions discussed in the section on usership in Chapter 2. Thus a medical device may be developed after implementation in the healthcare practice setting. These notions of flexibility versus the constraining parameters of irreversibility in innovation pathways will be key to my analysis of the medical device case studies through this book.

Governance and evidentiality

The intervention of the state is required to deal with 'market failure' in provision of healthcare generally and medical technologies in particular. It is useful to distinguish between broadly collective – state – and broadly market-like forms of provision of technologies (Rose and Blume, 2003). The case of technologies for medical application embraces both forms of provision. As Rose and Blume showed in the case of vaccination, different national states and healthcare systems may make available the same type of technology through different patterns of state/market arrangements. Thus in examining the transition of medical devices into healthcare systems, it is necessary to investigate the role of the state and the commercial marketplace in relation to sectors, zones and specific device technologies. Here, I briefly introduce some key concepts that are necessary to understand recent developments in the government activity associated with states, especially with the rise of 'neoliberal governance' across many societies globally. The most crucial concepts that I will consider here are those of the 'regulatory state', the 'health care state' and 'governance', distinct from and referring to a different formation of societal steerage than 'government'. The points to be made here are closely linked to the notion of the constructive force of regulatory policymaking in shaping and reshaping technological zones and industrial sectors. The rise of the evidence-based policy movements, which is integral to these developments in political agency, has become a crucial aspect of the governance of healthcare systems, which I will consider in the subsequent section. I use the term 'evidentiality' to refer to the phenomenon of the political movement towards evidence-based policy and practice in public sector services.

The growth of neoliberal governance over the last two decades has been characterised as involving a move away from command-and-control modes of direct government and service provision. It has a variety of distinctive features, including engagement of plural actors combining governmental, public institutional, private, voluntary, charitable and co-opted organisations, and groups interacting in both policy networks and looser 'issue networks' (Rhodes, 1997). A separation of standards and target-setting from operational, supply and delivery functions has been a widespread development. In particular, the move to less hierarchical management and control has opened a space in which has grown an increased emphasis on evidence-gathering and information-processing, and the use of information as a control mechanism (Majone, 1997). These global developments have been summarised, for example, as a 'reorientation of state policies toward deregulation, privatization and liberalization' (Haque, 2002). In such analysis, the nation state such as the UK may be conceptualised as the 'regulatory state' (Moran, 2001), orchestrating the agendas and activities of component agencies and networks around strategic objectives and performance targets. In relation to medical technology, however, constellations of governance relationships between stakeholders and social actors may be more or less fluid and fragile, and new strategic alliances between them *may* challenge established modes of governance (Fox et al., 2007). On the other hand, the resilience of medico-industrial institutionalised power structures in capitalist regulatory states may counter movements of active citizenship, for example in pharmaceutical technology (Abraham and Lewis, 2002).

The political economy of the European Union (EU) is important to the world of medical devices because of EU-wide regulatory regimes which define markets and the rules of engagement for trade in the European Economic Area (discussed in detail in Chapter 3). The jurisdiction of Europe is increasingly important as an arena for health policy and governance, more so in some aspects – such as public health and infectious disease – than others – such as medical care policy. Social theory and political science analysis point to the crucial part played by the harmonisation of standards within technological zones and political jurisdictions: the 'EU's governance blend ... requires European domains to be constituted in order that they may be governed' (Delanty and Rumford, 2005: 146). The Europeanisation of health policy is advancing, marked by a tension between 'deregulation and liberalisation' and 're-regulation and harmonisation' (Steffen et al., 2005). 'Europe' can be regarded as a site of the construction and negotiation of zones in which scientific and technological knowledge and goods may circulate, and such zones themselves are sites of the active application of regulatory standards. Technical standardisation is a *sine qua non* of technological zones (Callon, 2004). Thus in the case of medical devices and related technologies, the extent and nature of standardisation achieved through specific regulatory regimes is crucial to an understanding of both industrial economy and health protection through standards for the safety, quality and efficacy of devices entering the healthcare system.

The political economy of health and medicine in the regulatory state has also been developed in the notion of the 'health care state' (Moran, 1999). This concept draws attention to the deep interpenetration of healthcare institutions and government institutions, and the extension of healthcare politics outside the arena of healthcare. State and healthcare system are inextricably linked, and Moran's analysis shows how the healthcare state has become meshed with national industrial economy – the medical devices and pharmaceutical industries. The shift towards a governance-based model of control raises questions about alternative gatekeeping methods.

Closely integrated with the evolving governance formations in public services is the new evidentiality. It is clear that the scientific methods of healthcare evidentiality have emerged as one of the innovative gatekeeping regimes. The rise of the regulatory state, in national and European modes, and the movement from government to governance in which networks and enrolment between state and experts are key features, characterise significant developments in the relations of science, civil society and politics. In this environment the credibility of knowledge, or evidence, has become paramount. The growth of evidentiality represented by the new healthcare sciences can be understood as providing tools by which the state, the healthcare professions and medical technology industries may seek the social legitimation of healthcare innovation and governance. The case studies in this book provide some evidence about the constitution of such government-related gatekeeping activities, and some indications of their success. I turn to a brief discussion of evidentiality in the UK in the following section, highlighting developments which are relevant to the subsequent device-specific case studies presented in Chapters 4 to 8.

Healthcare science in the UK

The relationship between science and policy is a central concern in contemporary regulatory states. The importance of the link between governance and scientific evidentiality is increasingly recognised within professional networks of medicine. To give a trailer for the device technologies discussed in this book, in the controversial case of detection of localised prostate cancer:

> Stronger and braver governance is required to ensure that responsible decisions about risk management emerge for areas such as screening, which have such potentially enormous individual and societal consequences. These decisions must be based on sound research and proper partnerships.
>
> (Thornton and Dixon-Woods, 2002)

The rise of research-based evidentiality in healthcare accords with the widely documented move towards problem-oriented science.[2] The evolving modes of science are characterised by complexity, hybridity, non-linearity, reflexivity, heterogeneity and transdisciplinarity. Such 'post-normal' science reacts against the social segregation of expert knowledge from stakeholder and community participation. It is associated with complex 'unstructured' problems crossing traditional domains of enquiry and thus promoting transdisciplinary methodologies.

The new sciences of healthcare move in the direction of this post-normal science. This has been obvious in the huge scientific development in multidisciplinary Health Services Research (HSR) and Health Technology Assessment (HTA), which has been characteristic of government R&D policy in the UK and elsewhere, in pursuit of a 'knowledge-based health service'. The early development of the aims, disciplines, institutions, methodologies and epistemology of HTA in the UK have been described elsewhere (Faulkner, 1997; Harrison, 1998; Woolf and Henshall, 2000). These analyses highlight modernist quantitative, experiment-based and positivist methods, multidisciplinarity, linkage between scientific and policy institutions, and a focus on agendas of the effectiveness of healthcare interventions and cost-effectiveness. More lately, it is clear that additional approaches to methodology have gained ground, notably in the use of qualitative research methods associated with the social sciences, and in a greater attention to issues of patients' experiences of healthcare and health technologies. The quest to improve the theory and methodology of HTA continues (see, for example, Battista, 2006).

National institutions of healthcare evidentiality have been developed, and have been accorded a high degree of authority within healthcare policy. Newly designed institutions, such as the NHS Centre for Reviews and Dissemination and the National Institute for Health and Clinical Excellence (NICE) in the UK, can usefully be seen as boundary organisations acting to promote the generation and processing of healthcare science in the service of policy. Most obviously, these institutions lay claim to credibility through processes of centralisation. This applies both to the processes by which evidence is brought together and summarised, in particular through the use of systematic review methodology, and to the institutions' organisational forms as symbolic national centres. The scientific production of evidence has become organised in an institutional context, which involves negotiating control over the boundary between the scientific and R&D worlds of innovation and the world of health service application. HTA has been developed as a form of *regulatory* science (Lehoux and Blume, 2000). In contrast to medical device regulation, HTA has been concerned primarily with control over the introduction and diffusion into the healthcare system of devices, which have already been approved and certified in terms of safety and biocompatibility.

NICE commissions its own 'technology assessments and technology appraisals', appraisals being designed to take account of societal and stakeholder interests, while assessments focus on the scientific evidence (cf. Gabbay and Walley, 2006). Decisions about guidance to the NHS on adoption policy for new pharmaceuticals or technologies are made by a select group of individuals. But the evidence they refer to and their interpretation of it can then be challenged by interested parties. Multi-stakeholder 'hearings' for the consideration of the evidence – now in both the 'scientific' and quasi-legal senses of the word – about particular new technologies are therefore part of the modus operandi of NICE. Thus, in NICE the scientific evidence of healthcare safety and effectiveness and cost-effectiveness of devices is brought together with the range of interests that stakeholders represent. Institutions such as NICE thus act as buffers between evidence-producers and evidence-consumers, allowing for 'the politics' of the products of healthcare science to be considered in the wider society; it functions to politicise the evidence. The status of HTA evidence and NICE's regulatory guidance for the healthcare system figure prominently in the case study analyses which I present in this book.

Social scientists and some practitioners of HTA have criticised NICE for its inability to consider social, ethical and legal aspects of technology diffusion, in spite of its claims to this agenda (Faulkner, 1997). This challenge to conventional boundaries has been expressed, for example, in calls to 'de-monopolise' the assessment paradigm of HTA (Webster, 2004a) by making policy networks more open to societal participation, and by arguments to focus clearly upon multidimensional methods of seeking societally 'desirable' technologies (Lehoux, 2006). One of my aims in this book, in the spirit of these critiques of HTA, is to set evidence of HTA-style device assessments alongside multidimensional analysis of the socio-economics of medical device innovation, in order to provide a broader picture of the complex, interrelated dynamics of material technology, innovation, societal assessment and governance.

This book tries to develop ways of understanding the material technology of medical devices in their patterned relationships with social, governance and evidential processes. Thus, for some devices the material technology and its episodes of intervention in the human body are, in themselves, of relatively little significance or concern. Blood tests administered by health professionals, for example, are largely innocuous, both physically and intellectually. However, the socially and professionally constructed interpretation of the data produced from blood tests is, of course, highly salient. Compare this to, say, artificial hip joints, where the device is embedded in the human skeleton and tissues. In this case, the artefact itself and the episodes of surgical intervention are key to the significance of the device in the healthcare context and in society.

This chapter has outlined key notions useful in understanding the dynamics of innovation, evidentiality and governance of medical technological development, and has summarised key aspects of the rise of scientific evidentiality in healthcare. I have emphasised concepts of forces structuring healthcare and society: the political economy, industrial sectors and technological zones, the regulatory state, innovation pathways, the scientific evidentiality movement. In the case studies of medical devices presented in this book, the formation and effects of these structuring forces will be analysed in detail. In examining the innovation pathways of the device technologies, societal and healthcare actors are conceived of as stakeholders pursuing interests at the articulation points of innovation and governance. The concept of stakeholder interests raises questions regarding the patterning of relationships between different actors involved in shaping medical device technologies and their innovation into healthcare practice. In order to tackle these questions, it is useful first to examine some of the concepts of society/technology dynamics developed in a range of social science studies over the last 20 years or so. This is the subject of the next chapter.

2
Approaching Technology

Contemporary healthcare is technological healthcare. An adequate understanding of how medical technologies reach the healthcare system, and in what forms, must pay due attention to the activity of industrial sectors and political regulatory activity, as well as actors in the healthcare system, patients and citizens whose lives are touched by technology. In order to approach the issue of medical device innovation into healthcare, I here consider research and theory in the social sciences, which has developed a range of concepts and theoretical approaches that can be applied to the world of medical devices. This will pave the way for the main theme of this book, which is to understand the key social and evidential dynamics in the innovation pathways into healthcare of different medical devices.

The conundrum of society/technology

The relationship between society and technology is by now the subject of a very substantial body of theoretical analysis and empirical research in the social sciences. In order for this book to delve into the world of medical devices and healthcare innovation, it will be useful first of all to take some bearings in the broad universe of society/technology studies. Here, therefore, I describe what I take to be some of the key insights from this field, in order to approach the world of medical devices armed with appropriate conceptual tools. It is important to highlight some of these society/technology concepts for the discussion of medical devices that I present here, because I aim to show how the patterns of social-technological causation differ for different device technologies. My starting point is thus that there is unlikely to be a satisfactory one-size-fits-all society/technology theory. The final sections of Chapters 4 to 8 in this book consider the devices in terms of society/technology studies, and a comparative analysis of the five case studies is presented in Chapter 9.

In Chapter 1, I introduced concepts of state governance and the evidence movements as forces in the shaping of medical technology. Here the primary approaches that I briefly consider are, broadly, the 'social shaping' of technology, 'co-construction' of technology and society and 'technology-in-practice'. The scale of these areas of study has grown to such an extent over the last 20 years that it is impossible to survey them comprehensively. My aim is to highlight some of the key insights and concepts that can be useful tools with which to approach the world of medical devices and healthcare innovation.

First, however, it will be helpful to sound a note of warning about terminology. I am using the combined terminology of 'society/technology', which is intended to convey the close proximity of the concepts and the close empirically observable (or at least deducible) dynamics between particular technologies and particular manifestations of societal processes. My sense of the conundrum of society/technology causality is that while it is often the case that society/technology should be understood as denoting inextricably interlinked processes, it is nevertheless sometimes useful in analysing particular cases to treat the social and the technological 'as if' they are separate spheres. Thus if one wishes to explain, for example, the rise to prominence of the technology of X-ray equipment, attention to various 'social' actors – industrial, medical, business, hospital and so on – will be appropriate. Equally, attention to various 'technological' processes and entities such as electromagnetic radiation, tungsten, electrons and photographic plates will be required. On the other hand, if the aim is to make theoretical generalisations about how the design of X-ray machines has come to be the way that it is, or about how they are used in everyday diagnostic practices, one might wish to say that we can understand them as a 'sociotechnology' or as constituting a set of 'sociotechnical' practices.

A second note of warning is that I treat 'technology' and medical device technologies as referring primarily to physical materials and manufactured artefacts. And beyond physical artefactuality *per se*, both the design and development, and the deployment or active consumption of technologies, are achieved by social actors applying various expertise, techniques, skills, knowledge and methods. There are, of course, some technological applications where the artefactual, 'hard' definition is not easy to maintain, the obvious example being the information and communication technologies (ICTs) where the substantive action is the manipulation of digital information in 'computerised' forms. However, by and large I will stick to the artefactual definition. In this field, the use of the term 'technology' is often deployed with a much broader meaning than this. Thus some well known formulations of technology, such as Michel Foucault's widely adopted notion of 'technologies of power' and 'technology of the self', in which structured forms of social, organisational and institutional action are regarded as technologies (Foucault et al., 1988), or the less ideological 'social technologies' defined by their influence on human behaviour (Pinch et al., 1992), are outside the definition of technology to be used here. Equally excluded are broad characterisations of the extent to which technology as a generic phenomenon may be a defining and forceful feature of contemporary advanced industrial society – 'technological rationality' (Marcuse, 1964), 'technological society' (Barry, 2001) and technology of Europe (Callon, 2004).

I now turn to the key concepts of society/technology studies that are useful for approaching the world of medical devices and healthcare innovation.

Social shaping

An overriding concern in society/technology studies has been the direction of causal relationships between the social and the technological. In very broad terms, there has been a reaction against the view that society merely responds to technological innovation – technological determinism. A landmark early work in this context was the book entitled *The Social Shaping of Technology* published in the mid-1980s (MacKenzie and Wajcman, 1985). As the editors of the book point out in its greatly revised second edition (1999), the approach to understanding society/technology that it embodied moved in the space of some 15 years from being something of a heresy to being 'almost an orthodoxy' (1999: xv). The insights of 'social shaping' are a necessary corrective to the determinism of much technology analysis that took the form of 'the impact of X on Y', where X is a technology, for example the telephone, and Y is an aspect of society, for example social networks. The simplified narratives of the history of technology abound with this sort of notion. Famously, for example, the stirrup was credited with bringing about the feudal system. It remains important to state and restate the value of a social shaping approach, not least because technological determinism frequently rears its head in everyday and mass media discourse about technologies. The message of social shaping is that technology is not a neutral, value-free, non-social force to which society simply responds.

Ever since the seminal notion of 'the social construction of reality' was formulated (Berger and Luckmann, 1967), social constructionism has become a pervasive force in the social sciences. In social studies of technology, a 'social construction of technology' (SCOT) was important in elaborating ways in which social processes might be involved in shaping the *design* and constitution of technologies – for example, different designs of bicycles and the different scientific groups with which the inventor of Bakelite interacted (Bijker, 1995; Bijker et al., 1987; Schwartz Cowan, 1987). These SCOT studies were focused on the technology-producer and technology-user relationships in the free marketplace, so not generally maintaining a view of a particular *sector* of human activity such as is represented by medicine and healthcare. In the case of medical devices, it is clear that in spite of the great diversity of technologies involved, healthcare and medical systems and their participants act as institutional frames that mediate the development and adoption of new technologies. The SCOT approach has been subject to two main critiques of omission which are relevant to the multi-dimensional approach to medical technology that I develop in this book. Firstly, it has been noted widely that the approach is both design-focused and artefact-centric, thus neglecting processes of development and engagement with users (e.g. Hyysalo, 2004: 41) and secondly, it has been criticised from the outset and more recently for its inattention to matters of social structure, power relations and political and industrial economy (for example, Russell and Williams, 1988; Klein and Kleinman, 2002). As noted in Chapter 1, it is necessary to attend to both, to usership of technology and to matters of governance in examining innovation in the medical device and healthcare sector.

Combining different approaches (including historical), an early 1990s study, recognising a measure of alignment with social constructionist approaches, gave a detailed analysis of the participants in the development of diagnostic imaging technologies, including the contribution of clinical actors (Blume, 1992). Blume concluded, against the grain of theories either of evolutionary technological determinism or of capitalist industrial domination, that a driving force was the symbiotic and negotiated *integration* of medical and industrial interests in which neither was especially dominant. This is highlighted in a later study discussing collective – state – and market-like forms of provision of vaccine technologies (Rose and Blume, 2003). Thus it is important to consider the market/state relationship in technology innovation and governance in any sector.

Engineering

It is useful also to consider how actors in the worlds of technological development may be characterised. A key constructionist concept here has been that of 'heterogeneous engineering' (Law, 1987). The usefulness of this notion lies in its highlighting of the nature of the work that is performed by the designers, developers and producers of technologies. At heart, the notion is simple: engineers' work engages not only with technical materials, design concepts, calculation and so on, but it engages also with social process. Thus technological engineering is at the same time societal engineering. Engineers are 'heterogeneous' in bringing together and negotiating not only materials and designs but also social actors such as interest stakeholders, social institutions and users or potential users. Thus here the social process includes also the envisioning and creation of markets for technologies, where the formation of markets is considered as a process by which the economy itself is shaped, at least partly, by the proponents of technology. Heterogeneous engineering, therefore, points, albeit not very explicitly, towards the relationships of power and resources between social actors in the production and deployment of technologies.

A further development of the 'heterogeneity' concept of technology is that technological products amount to a network of juxtaposed components constituted from the interplay of a disparate array of elements, both social and 'technical'. This concept drew upon the notion of the interdependent 'network' in a historian's account of electrification (Hughes, 1983). Thus Law's analysis raised questions about the 'socialness' and materiality of actors that shape technology's innovation pathways.

Co-construction and technology-in-practice

The concept of a network of actors has been developed in notions of the 'co-construction', 'co-production' or 'co-constitution' of technology and society. This concept is difficult to fault. Society shapes technology; technology shapes society; the components of each interact with the others. However, like social shaping, this concept in its highly generalised form obscures more than it reveals. It is used in many formulations as a form of shorthand for what should be seen as complex relationships between the social and the technical in particular instances. Thus in this book I argue for the need to develop understandings of device innovation pathways that acknowledge *asymmetrical* relationships between social actors and healthcare artefacts, if and where they are found.

The concept of co-construction requires that we consider the theoretical approach of actor-network theory which conceptualises material technology as an 'actor' in networks of interacting agents (for example, Law and Hassard, 1999). While accepting, as a general principle, that 'artefacts have politics' (Winner, 1985) in their design and implementation, we can ask, in the world of medical devices: 'do devices have stakes'? Following the early theorisation of SCOT, it is clear that manufactured devices have material qualities that do interact in *more* or *less* flexible ways with social actors. Thus the 'obduracy' (Bijker, 1995) of materials and artefacts is a force in networks of interacting con-stituencies that shape healthcare device innovation processes. As bat-tery cells were actors in the (non-) evolution of the electric car in France (Callon, 1986), the particular electronic, software design features and material components of, say, infusion devices, are forces that impinge on their usage possibilities, adoption patterns and diffusion routes in healthcare settings. Equally, these technological characteristics are 'socially shaped' by the goals, design concepts and material innovations of actors in the medical device industries.

Many studies that embrace a social shaping or co-construction per-spective tend towards a rather inflexible reductionism. From an *a priori* perspective, I expect that any given technology determines social rela-tions and social experience more than others; conversely, in some cases 'society' determines technological developments more than others. The conclusion from these considerations is, first, that only empirical stud-ies will enlighten us as to which type of formulation is most apt in a given case, and, second, that we must be careful when deploying high-level concepts which try to capture the *general* direction of power and influence in society/technology relations.

While the society/technology concepts discussed above do entertain notions of the *users* of technology, the emphasis tends to be upon *design* and the social and technical processes that produce the technology. An alternative to technological determinism and 'social essentialism' has been summarised as a 'technology-in-practice' approach (Timmermans and Berg, 2003a). Apart from being closely aligned with co-construction, this approach makes the case, applied to society/technology studies of medicine, for focusing our attention on the more 'invisible' and mun-dane technologies. In healthcare, this approach should focus upon technologies such as 'records, information systems, standards, small home-care technologies' (op. cit., p. 108). The embedding of technology in 'tools, practices, groups, professionals, and patients' (p. 104) encap-sulates a notion of the inextricability of society/technology relations.

Hence, here we are taken deep into what I will term the *usership* of technologies, the way in which they become embedded in everyday professional and patient practices, their social meanings and their implications for social organisation in the workplace and elsewhere.

This technology-in-practice focus, and actor-network theory, has little room for theoretical approaches built on notions such as social structure or political economy or even capitalism (cf. Mackenzie, 1999). In Chapter 1, I discussed concepts such as 'innovation systems' and the 'healthcare state' that do permit analysis of the direction of technological change in terms of 'structural' socio-economic shaping forces. In spite of the claim that the common thread in technology-in-practice is that ethnographic or historical analysis investigates 'the practice of designing or using' the technology, in fact it appears that most studies are focused upon usership rather than design and the political economy in which design processes are embedded.

A focus on the *usership practices* of technology is a useful one and raises a number of important issues: how are people constructed as device users, or how do social actors make themselves into users? How do different social constituencies (for example, surgeons, nurses, clinical engineers, designers, 'human factors' engineers, hospital risk managers, regulators, medical patients, citizens) interact to create patterns of usership of a particular technology? How does usership interact with design to *change* technologies? What are the structural forces shaping usership? These will be key questions in the case studies in this book, and in the section below I explore some of the key notions about usership that can be taken from sociological and science and technology studies.

Usership and citizenship

Much theorising about sociological approaches to technology discusses technologies as having been black boxed so that they are impervious in the social processes of their use. The power relationships, organisational structures and skill-sets that are embedded into and around technologies take on the appearance of solid, sometimes oppressive, locked-in realities. The *usership* of technology may thus be seen as overdetermined by 'upstream' processes of design and development, often in the hands of commercial industrial enterprises. This assumption lies behind much of the illuminating sociological and socio-historical work described above, focused upon the constructionist approach to understanding how technologies have come to be designed and used as they are.

Particularly influential here has been the concept of 'configuring the user' (Woolgar, 1991), which highlighted the ways in which usability studies conducted by information technology developers built up constraints on the scope of users' action. While the concept of black boxing has been useful in stimulating social constructionist approaches to society/technology, it is not always the case that technologies *are* straightforwardly black boxed and thus impervious to users' and wider society's interference and reshaping. Some may be more black boxed at the point of purchase or adoption than others. To anticipate the case studies in this book, in the world of medical devices it is common for medical practitioners such as surgeons to act as consultants in the design and development of particular devices. It is also the case that healthcare providers play an important role in the *application* of device technologies, and in some cases, such as testing technology for prostate cancer discussed in this volume, this may be more salient for society and for users – patients or citizens – than the material technology itself. Device developers and manufacturers may 'own' knowledge about device *use*, and will promote it in the healthcare marketplace. This issue of privatised knowledge and skills is taken up in several of my case studies.

Much of the sociological analysis of technology, therefore, has been concerned with the ways in which and extent to which a technology's users and non-users might be active participants in shaping the design and deployment of technological products. A number of concepts have been proposed that point in this direction. For example, a focus on consumption (Schwartz Cowan, 1987) drew attention to the consumer as an active choice maker in a marketplace of competing technologies; understanding of the choice making required knowledge of consumers' everyday experience of social and technical networks. This perspective was a useful corrective to histories of technology that focused primarily upon 'upstream' invention, design and technology-push. Recent research here has included users and non-users as key participants in processes of technological innovation (Oudshoorn and Pinch, 2003). As Lehoux noted of this relationship in the case of healthcare, 'the extent to which health technology designers are truly knowledgeable about health care practices is a matter of considerable debate' (Lehoux, 2006: 75). And, one might add – doubt. In the same spirit of interrogating patterns of society/technology relations, questions have been raised about the *extent* to which users may 'fit' the imagined configurations that technology producers may have built up for them, and how users' actions may 'solidify, modify or reject' those configurations (Rose and Blume, 2003).

There has thus been a concerted effort in society/technology studies to find examples of how users have reshaped or found new uses for artefacts, undreamt of by their original producers. Pinch, for example, gives the example of the reinvention of record turntables as musical instruments for 'scratching' in DJ and other musical performances (Pinch, 2003). Akin to this notion of reinvention, a concept of 'domestication' has been outlined to point to the constructive processes with which consumers may engage with technologies, a process that may be influenced by commercial interventions: 'Field sellers are the active agents of how a technology is domesticated' (Pinch, 2003: 248). In the case of the medical device and pharmaceutical industries, the effect of marketing and the role of user modification are clearly important, though under-researched topics.

The theme of reinvention by users and the counter-expertise of citizens has been taken up in studies of innovation in medical technology. Much has been written about these instances of technological innovation in biomedicine where non-institutionalised experts have emerged from the citizenry and had an impact upon established expertise and innovatory practice. The so-called 'AIDS activists' in the US are one of the most often-quoted examples (Epstein, 1996; Epstein, 2000). This account shows how gay citizens in the US were able to gain sufficient technical expertise in order to challenge prevailing standards and practices for the conduct of clinical trials of new drugs under the regulatory regimes of the Food and Drug Administration (FDA). Even more radical in terms of 'citizen science' (Irwin, 1995) has been the growth in technological research and development in which 'concerned' citizens have been the prime movers, directly involved in shaping research agendas (Rabeharisoa and Callon, 2002; Callon and Rabeharisoa, 2003) and becoming patent holders (Novas, 2006). Contrasted to these forms of active citizen engagement in technology innovation, are examples of active resistance – *non-use* – of the products of technological medicine. A notable example here is that of cochlear implants (Blume, 1995 and 1997). Promoted as a 'cure' for profoundly deaf people, especially children, activists from deaf communities have mobilised in many countries in order to resist the social diffusion of the device.

What might be called the 'users-as-designers' approach, taken to its logical extreme, results in an analysis that collapses the 'artificial divide between design and use' (Oudshoorn and Pinch, 2003). While the divide between design and use may be artificial if one is attempting to produce a general theory of agency in technology innovation, obscuring as it may do interactions between end-users and design processes, to jettison the distinction entirely may be counterproductive. A co-constructivist formulation such as 'design-use' runs the risk of obscuring more than it reveals, and again this points to the need to examine patterns of design-user interaction in shaping device technologies in particular instances. Although healthcare systems such as that in the UK are increasingly marketised, the market is well known to be dissimilar to commercial direct-to-consumer marketplaces in various ways: patients may lack knowledge to make purchasing decisions; the medical profession traditionally acts as an expert intermediary, and for *many* devices this continues to be the case; clinical collectives tend to develop conventional beliefs and practices that shape procurement strategy; the state of evidence of safety, risk, benefit and effectiveness may conflict with producers' ambitions. Much of the usership of device technologies is mediated by healthcare professionals and purchasing organisations and state-orchestrated policymaking. However, this should not blind us to instances where the citizen-patient is, or could be, the direct user of a device. The important question here remains: *which* devices/technologies may be more or less susceptible to users' participation, under what circumstances, and why?

Engineering design itself, of course, includes a number of approaches to usership in its methodologies. Most obviously, this includes ergonomics-based approaches and 'usability testing'. However, there are more radical approaches to the attempted incorporation of users into design and development processes. A notable example in the UK is part of an innovative research programme that attempts to develop upstream methods of valuing future device technologies, including user participation in the innovation process (MATCH, 2007; Ram et al., 2005; Shah and Robinson, 2007).

In summary, it may be that some technologies are more 'configurable' in society/technology relations than others, as the concept of obduracy suggests. Equally, some technologies more than others may have different flexibilities of 'affordance' (Hutchby, 2001) of social organisation. Questions of whether and how people interacting with medical devices are configured or configure themselves as 'users' or as citizens or as patients, in relation to different technologies, are highlighted in the case studies in the book. I now consider the issue of flexible configurability of technologies by way of a short discussion of typologies of technology that sociologists and organisational analysts have devised.

Typologies of technology

Different technologies may evoke different patterns and powers of usership, and users of technologies may domesticate, adapt, or innovate technologies in ways that are constrained by characteristics of a technology itself. Scholars in this field have made a number of illuminating distinctions between types of technology, which are relevant to the case studies of medical device discussed in this book.

The notion of *complexity* figures large in conceptualisations of society's attempts to manage contemporary technology. In the notion of 'normal accidents', for example, high-risk technologies (socio-technical systems such as nuclear power stations and chemical processing plants) have been distinguished along two dimensions (Perrow, 1999). Firstly, 'loosely-coupled' and 'tightly-coupled' technologies are identified, and secondly, 'complex' and 'linear' technologies (Perrow, op. cit.). In tightly coupled technologies, the interaction between parts or flows in a sequence are compact, dynamic, closely interdependent and usually fast or difficult to intervene in. Complex technologies are characterised not only by multiple internal components, but also by widely varying processes, interactions and connections, contributing materials and practices and flows that have knock-on effects. In an insight highly relevant to medical devices and device-rich environments (and in an insight that has echoes of Beck's risk society hypothesis (1992)), Perrow notes that the development of safety systems may, in fact, compromise safety – by increasing the overall level of complexity.

The concepts of complexity and coupling may appear in different guises in other typologies. Molina, influenced by the 'social shaping' approaches discussed above, has reviewed technology-centred typologies, albeit in the context of industrial economy rather than healthcare systems (Molina, 1999). Distinctions of product/process and assembled/non-assembled are rather narrow descriptions applicable to industrial process and products, whereas 'infrastructural', 'informational' and 'open-ended' are broader and may include dynamics of technological interaction with society more broadly. Important here is a four-way schema of discrete technologies, component technologies, generic system technologies and configurational technologies (Fleck, 1994). Discrete technologies function as self-contained packages requiring no interfacing with other elements. Discrete technologies, in terms of innovation pathways, do not require the active participation of users in their day-to-day implementation. Component technologies are defined by their assembly by developers or manufacturers into a functional system, microprocessors being a good example. 'Generic system technologies', closer to the concepts of 'complex' and 'infrastructure' (e.g. electricity, railway-like) technologies, 'refer to complexes of elements or component technologies which mutually condition and constrain one another, so that the whole complex works together' (Fleck, op. cit., p. 18).

'Configurational' technologies, at the other end of the continuum, might be systems in early stages of evolution, or systems that are open-ended and flexible in their set-up. Each implementation is more or less unique. Configurational technologies typically include, for example, information and communication technology-based applications. In healthcare, telemedicine or telecare systems would be configurational technologies. In these technologies, significant innovation/configuration can be made by users in the process of implementation, and such processes may be regarded as learning processes (Fleck, 1994). A politico-sociological perspective may see processes of professional and sectoral contestation at work, rather than 'learning' (May et al., 2001).

The social shaping, co-construction/technology-in-practice and 'usership'-based approaches described above can be summarised as all depending on an actor or agency-based conception of society and the material world. As noted in the discussion on the social construction of technology, there is overall, in these approaches, a lack of study of the political and economic structure when it comes to Science & Technology Studies (STS) investigation of medical device technologies. Analysis of structural matters of political and industrial economy has been largely absent, not wholly surprisingly, given medical sociology's traditional focus on the medical consultation and interaction between patients and medical professionals. While there is some such analysis from the discipline of political science (e.g. Moran, 1999; Steffen, 2005 – both noted in Chapter 1), there is a clear need to address this weakness with empirically based analysis. The overview in this chapter, and analysis in this book highlights the need to understand the powerful structuring forces that affect 'the *capacity* of social groups to shape a technology' (Klein and Kleinman, 2002).

The field of study of medical technology/society innovation should thus pursue methods that combine attention to political economy and the medical sociologist's more traditional qualitative analysis of the social meanings of medicine (Conrad, 2005). In order to tackle such a programme, it is necessary to examine concepts that might be developed to assess the politico-economic forces that guide innovation pathways of technologies. I have drawn attention to some of these in Chapter 1, and here, firstly, I note the continuing salience of the concept of 'medicalisation' as a tool for understanding the conundrum of society/technology in the medical sphere, and secondly, I introduce the concept of 'technological zone' (Barry, 2001 and 2006) as a possible tool for enabling the macro- or meso-level (Swan et al., 2007) constraining and enabling forces on technology innovation to be brought into the foreground.

Medicalisation revisited

Medicalisation is a well known concept with a very long history in medical sociology. Here I want to draw attention briefly to recent developments and refinements of the concept that are relevant for a discussion of medical devices – in healthcare – in society. I do not recap the history of the concept or sociological research in this field; its several variants have been usefully outlined and discussed elsewhere (Ballard and Elston, 2005). These authors emphasise that medicalisation in contemporary societies should be seen as a more 'complex, ambiguous and contested' process than early formulations based around medical dominance allowed. In particular, medicalisation may or may not be seen as a social benefit. For example, there has been resistance to the medicalisation of childbirth, but rather less to the medicalisation of depression. Citizen-patients in many instances have become more active participants in extending medical care in certain conditions, as evidenced by patient advocacy and self-help groups. There are also, of course, examples of *de*medicalisation (for example, homosexuality) and anti-medicalisation (for example, cochlear implants, Blume, 1997, as noted in the discussion of usership above). The movement towards 'self-care' in health *may* be regarded as demedicalisation – I discuss the ambivalences in this interpretation in the case study of home-based therapeutic monitoring technology in Chapter 7. The point of this brief summary is that it is useful to conceive these developments of society/technology relations *in terms of* medicalisation, and that medicalisation is useful as a hypothesis with which to investigate the social relations of specific medical practices or technologies.

The second point of significance about medicalisation is its linkage with trends in the production and organisation of medicine/healthcare. Given the starting point that healthcare is technological healthcare, medicalisation may be technological medicalisation. Thus, we can hypothesise that technologically mediated medicalisation, or demedicalisation, may be a phenomenon of contemporary healthcare systems and medical professional practices in their interrelations with medical device and other bio-industries and the healthcare state. Such reconceptualisations of medicalisation have been argued notably by scholars in the US (Conrad, 2005; Clarke et al., 2003). Thus in the case studies of medical devices in this book I discuss medicalisation/demedicalisation in the significance of each technology as part of healthcare innovation and as part of broader social processes.

Technological zones

'Technological zone' as a concept may enable matters of structure (political economy, industrial organisation, innovation networks) to be brought together with the approaches to socio-technical innovation which are founded on a presumption of agency, whether the agents be individuals, collectivities, human or material. The term was introduced by Barry (2001). A technological zone is defined by the linked circulation and interaction of materials, knowledge, property and people rather than by given geographical, political or institutional boundaries with which they may or may not coincide – Barry gives high energy physics as an example where activity is both highly concentrated institutionally and highly dispersed geographically, and has also applied it to the oil industry. In a later development of the concept, Barry (2006) identifies three forms of technological zone, associated especially with the development of standardisation and common measurement methodologies that become shared between the diverse participants in zones. I do not attempt a detailed exploration or critique of the concept here[1], but adopt it as loosely applicable to the organisation of technology fields such as subgroups of medical devices and, in particular, tissue engineering (discussed as the final case study in this book). It is preferable to, for example, industrial 'sector', which has connotations of multiple technologies, stable institutional interdependencies, rules of engagement and product-based classifications (cf. Malerba, 2004). Sectoral concepts may be applicable to established industrial groupings but are inappropriate in the case of more emergent and unstable politico-economic and technological change such as tissue engineering.

3
The World of Medical Devices

Introduction

The world of medical devices is a complex, fragmented and paradoxical one. Its boundaries and contours are difficult to delineate, its societal participants not always obvious or easy to discern, its rules of engagement variable and contested, information about it relatively difficult to obtain, its technologies multiple and interdependent, its technology classifications labyrinthine and bureaucratic. In short, from the perspective of wider society, the world of medical devices is obscure. Paradoxically however, as citizens we are surrounded by this world and its particularities, and we interact with it by a multitude of routes in our daily lives, in sickness and in health. Medical devices enter into our intimate and family relationships, into our understandings of health and disease, our values and beliefs, our practices of looking after our own health, as well as our experience of healthcare systems and healthcare professionals' work.

It is unlikely that many individuals live their lives without encountering one or other medical device. Some individuals will experience hundreds of them. They exist in massive numbers, shapes, sizes, materials and designs. Some single device types, heart pacemakers for example, may have hundreds of different models available to the end-user. Technological innovation is endemic, ranging from slight variants or modifications to existing devices, to some breakthrough technologies. Via biotechnology, more and more hybrid device technologies are being developed, as in the case of tissue engineering. The advanced healthcare systems are simply inconceivable without a myriad array of different device technologies. Yet many people will encounter medical devices without realising their connection with the processes of industrial capitalism, governmental policy,

27

structures of healthcare delivery and consumption, scientific evaluation of safety and effectiveness, medicalisation and technological innovation.

That medicine is becoming increasingly technological (and biotechnological) is irrefutable, and the pace of the change is accelerating. The concept of 'technology' dominates sociological and anthropological thinking, rather than 'device'. But if we are to understand processes of innovation of medical devices into healthcare systems, then we should consider the ways in which the technologies of medicine are framed within contemporary society. Thus, notably, technologies are framed as 'medical devices' as part of industrial activity and by regulatory regimes. This chapter outlines the significance of these two sectoral forces. It should be noted that the nomenclature of 'device' is not shared across all regulatory or policy arenas. Thus the important activity of HTA, discussed here as healthcare evidentiality, frames medical devices as one group of 'health technology' alongside pharmaceuticals, surgical procedures and organisational and other healthcare interventions.

In this chapter, I note technical trends in medical device technology and describe the nature of the industry and market and innovation processes in the sector. I outline important aspects of the emergence and operation of medical device regulation in Europe and the UK. I also note some developments in UK innovation/regulation policies that will be referred to in the case studies of device-specific governance processes (Chapters 4 to 8). At the end of the chapter, I introduce the comparative case studies of medical devices in which the book's themes are developed and illustrated.

Material technology of medical devices

Medical devices encompass therapeutic, diagnostic, screening, inert and powered technologies. There are a number of contemporary technical trends affecting the material development of device technologies, and of course other technological arenas, at the beginning of the twenty-first century. The most notable of these include the incorporation of information and telecommunications technologies – the increasing embedding of software into devices, increasing use of electronic communication between devices in use and 'servers' and their host organisations; miniaturisation in general; and many developments associated with the advance of biomaterials and biotechnology. The latter include, for example, the introduction of bioactive coatings for orthopaedic implants and, especially, the increasing development of 'combination products' in which elements of devices are combined with pharmaceutical or biological technologies.

The advent of tissue engineering, discussed at length in the penultimate chapter of this book, is a development that challenges radically the conventional boundaries between the worlds of medical device and pharmaceutical. Nanotechnologies, also, are likely in the future to be an integral feature of device-based diagnostics and therapeutics, as well as pharmaceuticals. Technological innovation creates pressure for innovation into clinical use. Seductive visions of technological progress are typical of pressures that healthcare policymakers face and which industry policymakers support. Material innovation is endemic to medical devices, especially where perceived markets are large.

Deviceness and device classifications

When is a medical device not a medical device? Classification is at the heart of human sense making and purposeful social action. As Mary Douglas and other anthropologists argued many decades ago, classification processes are central to processes of making and remaking social institutions and to the development of societal meanings and values. Typologies are useful to the social scientist attempting to make society intelligible, and they are useful to healthcare actors – the medical profession, industry and its promoters and regulatory policymakers. Their respective typologies of medical technology rarely coincide closely. The structuring work of classification is particularly striking in the socio-medical and industrial worlds of medicine and healthcare (Bowker and Star, 1999). Classifications can usefully be seen as maps to the world of medical devices. Processes of classification of medical devices are part of society's regulatory ordering of innovating technological zones. Society's classifications of technology, as in other arenas, have important consequences for how risks and benefits are perceived, constructed and managed; what regulatory and evidential regimes are brought into play; what private or public resources might be deployed and what characteristics might be highlighted in the public sphere and thus give rise to public approval or concern.

It is important to recognise the significance of the ordering of socio-technological boundaries for regulation of technological sectors and zones such as in vitro diagnostics or tissue engineered technologies, as discussed here. This is especially the case in the era of biotechnology where the boundaries between technological/regulatable boundaries are increasingly threatened and undermined by innovation and hybridisation. Thus the boundaries of 'deviceness' in the world of biotechnology become a matter for negotiation and contestation (hip prostheses, for example, may include bioactive coatings; tissue engineering challenges the boundaries between pharmaceuticals and device technologies). The fluid boundaries between different categories of medical technology and healthcare products are continually being renegotiated, attacked and defended. Some medical technologies are framed by stakeholders as more 'devicey' than others. The chapter on tissue engineering in this book discusses some of the complexities of classificatory boundary making that are highlighted when regulatory and industrial forces meet around novel types of technology.

Attempts to devise systems for grouping and classifying device technologies may serve a variety of purposes. Here I discuss attempts by theorists to conceptualise the range and nature of device technologies and related classificatory systems, which are always evolving and subject to contestation by stakeholders, developed to 'underpin' the processes by which society appraises the acceptability of devices for human use. It will be seen also that regulatory classifications do not match the classifications used in industrial policy to segment and sectorise the healthcare products industries. Such classificatory systems become, to a greater or lesser extent, wired into the regulatory regimes by which national and transnational bodies such as the EU seek to promote and control the interfaces of technoscience, healthcare and society. At the most basic level it is such classifications that may distinguish between medicines, medical devices, biological treatments, blood and blood products, tissue banks and other therapeutic groupings.

The global and other transnational dimensions of medical devices are reflected in the social institutions that are now involved in their classification, promotion and regulatory governance. The World Health Organization, for example, has published a 'global overview' and guidance on medical devices (World Health Organization, 2003). This document advises governments internationally to 'follow the growing movement towards harmonized regulatory systems because a proliferation of different national regulations increases costs, hinders access to health care technologies, and can even unwittingly jeopardize the safety of the patient' (2003: vi). The WHO refers to the Global Harmonization Task Force (GHTF) (a global forum in which national device regulators meet) which states that a medical device 'means any instrument, apparatus, implement, machine, appliance, implant, *in vitro* reagent or calibrator, software, material or other similar or related article' used in healthcare, and not working by 'pharmacological, immunological or metabolic means' (in other words, not a drug) (World Health Organization, 2003) (see GHTF document SG1/N029R11).

The European Commission (EC) also has published guidance on the classification of medical devices. The risk-related philosophy underlying this is:

> A simple set of classification rules ... is impossible, because of the vast number and the changing nature of variables involved ... a classification concept which is essentially based on potential hazards related to the use and possible failure of devices taking account of technology used and of health policy considerations. This approach in turn allows the use of a small set of criteria that can be combined in various ways: duration of contact with the body, degree of invasiveness and local vs. systemic effect.
>
> (EC DG Enterprise, 2001: 3)

This results in groupings, not mutually exclusive, that include: devices with a measuring function, active devices, implantable devices and invasive devices. 'Active implantable' devices and 'devices for in vitro diagnosis' are separate groups again and in Europe are covered by separate legislative acts (Directives – see below). The European classification is closely tied to regulatory frameworks and legislative domains, which might promote and govern technological activity.

The medical device industrial economy and marketplace

There is strong evidence of the close intermeshing of medical device industry and the healthcare state. A growing involvement of private sector activity in healthcare systems has been noted from a variety of perspectives, including the advent of biomedical and biotechnology-driven industry (e.g. Foote, 1992; Gadelha, 2003 and 2004). Analysts have deployed a variety of terms to capture this proximity: a 'health-industrial nexus', 'corporate health', 'medical-industrial complex' and 'Biomedical TechnoService Complex' (Clarke et al., 2003). Given the interdependence of healthcare delivery systems and device industries, it is useful to conceive of their relationship as occurring in the spheres of socio-economic production and market entry, and adoption and usership. Regulatory intervention occurs in both arenas as my case studies will demonstrate. In this book, while I assume the general validity of the 'nexus' forms of analysis, I am concerned through case studies to explore the extent and salience for healthcare adoption of such dynamics in specific technologies and device-specific configurations of production and usership.

The medical device industry is growing in importance and contribution to national economic productivity. It is impossible to know the number of different medical devices produced for the world's healthcare systems. The market is global, with high levels of import and export, but its global nature is highly unequal between different regions. The global sector includes a massive range of types of products. Estimates in the region of 10,000 device families and 400,000 different devices are not uncommon (EC DG Enterprise, 2006). The value of the global market was estimated at US$105 billion in 2001 (Furtado, 2001), but it has also been reported to be close to $200 billion, about half the size of the global pharmaceutical market, and growing steadily (DTI, 2005). The US accounts for some 43 per cent of the total market (DTI, 2006), Europe for over 20 per cent and the Asia-Pacific region for over 15 per cent. It is starkly clear that higher-income countries consume more medical devices. Estimation of the size of national economies in medical device sectors is difficult due to varying classification of the products and companies with diverse and multiple activity. The markets for medical devices are primarily national.

Within Europe, the new accession states consume less than the established 15 member states (Altenstetter, 2004). The UK medical device market represented a $5.5 billion market in 2005 (DTI, 2005), representing approximately 3 per cent of the global market. The UK's National Health Service (NHS) is said to be the largest single institutional customer for medical devices in the world. In the global view, and in a different classification system, Europe accounts for about 23 per cent of the total 'healthcare equipment and supplies' market. The European healthcare equipment and supplies market reached the value of $37.9 billion in 2004 (Datamonitor, 2005). Nearly half of this value was accounted for by surgical and medical instruments subsectors. Trade association Eucomed data on the European medical technology industry show that in 2005 medical technology sales in Europe amounted to €63.6 billion, an increase of 15 per cent since its previous report. Average expenditure on medical technology as a percentage of total expenditure in healthcare was estimated at 6.3 per cent in Europe (as against 5.5 per cent in the US – Eucomed, 2007c). The rate of growth (or decline) of different national markets is of course variable. For example, Datamonitor's analysis of Europe shows that in the years up to 2004 Germany's growth was relatively slow compared to France, Spain and the UK. The Asia-Pacific market is expected, from the mid-2000s, to grow at the fastest rate.

The leading companies in the sector in Europe include enterprises such as multiproduct health sector specialists Johnson & Johnson, the 3M Group, Baxter International (specialises in devices related to the blood and circulatory system including a major activity in renal therapy), Tyco International, GE Healthcare, Medtronic, Alcon and specialists in other sectors such as the electronics company, Siemens. There is specialisation among the largest companies. Medtronic is sometimes referred to as the world's leading medical technology company.

The United Kingdom healthcare equipment and supplies market represents about 12 per cent of the EU (EU-15) market and is reported to have grown by 7.4 per cent in 2005 to reach a value of $7854 million. Market analysts forecast that this market will have a value of $10,450 million in 2010, a major increase of 33 per cent from 2005 (Datamonitor, 2006). (Market value is defined as revenues generated through sales). The largest subsector within the UK market value is disposable devices such as syringes, catheters, electrodes, sutures, bandages, implantable prostheses and orthotics and prostheses. The UK market is said to have strong R&D capability, and it is especially strong in emerging sectors such as wound management and diagnostics (Datamonitor, 2006).

The UK is a net exporter in the medical device sector. The UK sector has over 2000 companies, of which around 85 per cent are small firms. Roughly 75 per cent of medical device activity in the UK is in the supply of medical and surgical equipment, with most of the rest made up of diagnostics product suppliers (*in vivo* and *in vitro*). The fastest growing areas include in vitro diagnostics, orthopaedics and advanced wound management – a particularly strong area for the UK, which represents 13 per cent of the global market (DTI, 2005). The sector directly employs in excess of 55,000 people, and sales of products and related services in the UK amount to about £6 billion. Exports are in the region of £3.5 billion. Sales in the UK market increased by about 17 per cent between 2000 and 2003. In the UK in 2001, 210 companies worked with electromedical equipment out of 2460 corporations in medical devices manufacturing (ABHI, 2002). The estimate of this sector's turnover in the UK in 1999 was £12.7. In the UK, local market size is seen as problematic by companies – only 3 per cent of the global market – so manufacturers are seen to need to reach other markets for their products (ABHI, 2002). Exports increased by 45 per cent during that period. R&D expenditure is around £325 million per annum.

Leading companies headquartered in the UK include: Huntleigh Technology which claims representation in over 120 countries

(Datamonitor, 2006); GE Healthcare provides medical imaging, medical diagnostics, patient monitoring systems, disease research, drug discovery and biopharmaceuticals services. The company is part of General Electric and is represented in more than 100 countries. Smith & Nephew focuses on four areas: orthopaedic reconstruction, orthopaedic trauma and therapies, endoscopy and wound management. It operates in 33 countries (website, 2005 data). The UK industry is highly fragmented due to the large number of product subsectors. Large US and German multinational conglomerates tend to dominate the UK market, with a considerable number of Small and Medium-sized Enterprises (SMEs) specialising in niche or 'boutique' equipment also having a significant presence.

Device innovation process

The medical technology industry structure contrasts with pharmaceuticals in that the majority of technological innovation occurs among SME companies. Major device companies frequently acquire early stage companies once a business model for their technologies has been stabilised. They improve the efficiency of producing the technology and use distribution networks for trading. Typically also, the large companies have a strategic aim of iterative improvement of the product through several product generations. The typical innovation pathway of medical devices thus involves 'postmarketing' usership feedback in building incremental developments of a device. This pathway may be regarded as a form of progress: 'Most novel medical technologies are launched with limited efficacy and performance data but this accumulates very rapidly and supports rapid iterative development of the product' (Padeletti, 2006). An example of the difference between medical technology and pharmaceuticals is in the area of treatment for slow heartbeat (bradycardia). In the mid-1970s a drug was introduced for this problem, around the same time as the first powered pacemakers were made available. Since that time there has been one new drug and over 150 iterations of pacemaker technology. The initial large and unwieldy device is now small, computerised and has e-connectivity (Padeletti 2006). It is estimated that the vast majority of devices, around 95 per cent, are incremental alterations to existing technologies. Hence the proliferation of variations on the same device within 'families'. As will be seen notably in the case study of artificial hips, even small variations to an existing design or component material may have large consequences for device performance.

The medical device–healthcare nexus in the UK

Evidence of an increasing integration among a nexus of interests of medical device industry and healthcare policy has been noted in the concept of the healthcare state in Chapter 1, and can be seen in recent developments in 'joined up' government policy. A recent far-reaching and highly influential review of the NHS addressed issues of medical technologies, stating that 'It is very clear that medical technologies have ubiquitous and profound implications for the delivery of healthcare in all health economies' (Wanless, 2002). It noted the 'slow and late adopter' status of the NHS, and suggested that this would be a 'cost and performance' problem for the NHS into the future if not addressed. A number of interrelated policy innovations initiated by the UK government are changing the innovation and adoption landscape for medical device technologies. In particular, following from the Wanless report, a UK government 'Healthcare Industries Taskforce' (HITF) was established, itself an innovative development in joining up between health policy and industry policy communities. This initiative brought together government and industry leaders to identify steps to maximise the benefit to patients of new and existing healthcare products.

The Healthcare Industries Taskforce expressed a need for the UK to contribute to shaping future device sectors, partly through regulatory regime-building:

> Engagement between Medicines and Healthcare products Regulatory Agency and industry on regulatory matters is fundamental and continuous. The HITF agenda has elevated the profile of this communication ... MHRA and industry have built on their existing excellent working relationship through a variety of stakeholder groups and regular discussions to draw up, agree, promote and secure UK objectives in important EU negotiations.
>
> (HITF, 2007)

Following from an HITF recommendation 'to forge closer links between product evaluation and purchasing' has been the decoupling of the former Device Evaluation Service from the Medicines and Healthcare products Regulatory Agency and its reconfiguring in the new form of the Centre for Evidence-based Purchasing (CEP) within the Purchasing and Supplies Agency of the NHS, in 2005. The importance of this move of nationally mandated technical device performance work from the pre-market/surveillance agency to the NHS procurement agency must be seen as a notable governance change. Its significance will be shown in the case studies of infusion pumps and artificial hips included in this book. A further attempt to 'join-up' different aspects of the healthcare device industry and regulatory regimes can be seen in the working of the Committee on the Safety of Devices, convened under the auspices of the MHRA. This committee, initiated as one of several national developments that have raised the profile of 'patient safety' as a focus for policy developments, has contributions from representatives of the Association for British Healthcare Industries (ABHI).

Other developments of significance for medical device innovation and healthcare adoption in the UK have been the replacement of the Modernisation Agency (1998–2005), which was the policy group that was the prime mover for process improvement in the NHS, by the NHS Institute for Improvement and Innovation, supported by regional 'Innovation Hubs'. The role of safety is promoted especially through the Health Care Commission and the new National Patient Safety Agency (NPSA). The latter is discussed in detail in the case study on infusion pumps.

Medical device regulation in Europe

The medical device industry has a stake in working towards the minimum possible number of entry points to international markets. Hence efforts at harmonisation across European countries are to the fore in European developments, and indeed 'global harmonisation' is the goal of a specific group, the Global Harmonization Task Force. The European Union has developed an approach to regulation of medical devices that is notably different from that of the US, the major market and industrial producer. After earlier measures targeting particular types of devices, three major legislative instruments of broad scope were introduced in the EU at intervals during the 1990s. These focus on three categories of technology: generic medical devices, 'active implantable' devices and 'in vitro diagnostic' devices. They deal with safety, efficacy and quality assessment for the placing of products on the market, and for a so-called vigilance system, which refers to the gathering and collation of 'postmarketing' data, in other words data about reported problems with devices following their introduction in the healthcare system. In accordance with the so-called 'New Approach to Harmonization', the European Medical Device Directive (MDD) of 1993 set out 'Essential requirements' for the approval process for medical devices. The twin aims of the directive were stated to be to promote trade and protect public health. Essential requirements apply to the design and construction of devices and must be shown to be met by the manufacturer. Under the directive a process of conformity assessment is required in order that manufacturers demonstrate compliance. The medical regulatory regime is administered through national 'competent authorities'. The designated competent authority for medical devices in the UK is the MHRA (Devices); this is the successor body to the previous Medical Devices Agency(MDA).

The essential requirements revolve around risk assessment–based classification of products. The directive set out guidance for the classification of devices according to their risk status on a four-point scale. Class I (for example, bandages) were those deemed to be the lowest risk and Class III the highest (for example, artificial heart valves and HIV tests). The intervening classes are known as Class IIa and Class IIb. The case studies in this book note the risk classification status of the devices in question. Devices may be subject to reclassification, although because of the legal framing of the regulation, this is a difficult and time-consuming process within the European system. The significance of reclassification is discussed in the chapter of this book on artificial hips, orthopaedic joints being one of the two most widely used and controversial devices whose risk classification has recently been upgraded (from class IIb to III), the other being another implantable device – the even more controversial breast implant (see Kent, 2003).

Different institutional regimes for the production of evidence, which may or may not include clinical data, apply to each risk class. These range from self-declaration by a manufacturer (often referred to as a 'self-certification' system) to a requirement that an independent expert must review the design, certify the manufacturing processes and/or test the finished product. For Class IIa devices the intervention of a notified body at the production stage is compulsory, whereas for devices in Classes IIb and III inspection by a notified body is required for the design and manufacture; for some Class I devices prior authorisation with regard to conformity is required for placing on the market. The organisations providing technical assessment are known as 'Notified Bodies' and are organised on a pan-European basis, meaning that a manufacturer in one country may apply to a body in any EU state where there is a body certified to have the appropriate expertise for the type of technology. Notified Bodies are usually private commercial companies mandated in the EU regulatory system, so in terms of contemporary governance they may be regarded as representing a form of 'regulated self-regulation'. The most obvious public evidence that a medical device is recognised under the EU system is the well known 'CE' mark

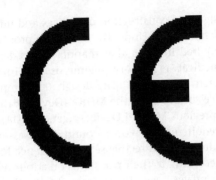

Figure 3.1   The CE-mark logo

(Conformité Européen; see Figure 3.1). If a product conforms to EU requirements, it will be CE-marked.

The European regulatory regime for devices does not necessarily require evidence of efficacy in clinical trials, or even the performance of new clinical trials. Evidence of mechanical performance in laboratory tests is sufficient for many new devices. This regime, therefore, is designed to assess whether a product is safe to use and 'fit for purpose'. A crucial consideration here is whether the product is deemed to be a 'new' product, or whether it is a copy or near-copy ('substantially equivalent') of a device already on the market. This concept is similar to the 'me-too' concept that is used in pharmaceutical innovation. Thus it is notable that the comparative effectiveness of a new product (whether it performs better in terms of patient outcomes) is not part of the pan-European regulatory regime. The comparative effectiveness issue is dealt with, if at all, primarily at national or local healthcare levels, as I have described above in discussing health technology assessment and healthcare evidentiality.

Apart from assessment of products for *entry* into the European marketplace, member states are required to establish vigilance systems for *post-marketing surveillance*. Manufacturers are required by law to report any serious incidents involving devices they produce or sell, and if they recall a particular type of device for technical or medical reasons. In the UK, the regulatory authority also operates an 'Adverse Incident Centre' to which users (for example, nurses, clinicians, patients) are able to report cases where a device has failed or produced unwanted side effects. This is a voluntary system. Following investigation by the regulatory authority, a number of actions may follow: *a hazard notice* may be issued alerting others to potential danger; *a safety notice* may be issued advising users in less urgent situations; or *a device bulletin* with guidance and information for users may be issued. Since January 2000, a *device alert* has been introduced where there is uncertainty about the potential for death or serious injury and where the medical device is likely to be implicated (MDA, 2001a). In some cases the manufacturer will withdraw the product from the market. Within the UK, the MDA/MHRA has a duty under the Consumer Protection Act, 1987, to enforce the essential requirements of the MDD regulations (MDA, 1995). The extent to which there is national variation in reporting procedures and policies is a matter for further empirical investigation (Faulkner and Kent, 2001), but the vigilance system is intended to allow sharing of data and information between competent authorities across Europe (MDA, 1998a).

In some countries national registries provide a means of tracking the use of certain types of devices. I will discuss the significance of this form of surveillance as part of device governance processes especially in the case study of artificial hips. The potential for expanding the use of registries was under discussion by the European parliament in the early 2000s (Black, 2001) and within the UK (DoH, 2000; RCS, 2001).

'Technical' standards are not mandatory. EU institutions have been set up to develop consensus agreements about technical standards for devices. This has produced harmonised European standards for some products. Under the European Commission DG Enterprise and Industry, the European Committee for Standardization (CEN) is the European body whose mission is to promote voluntary technical harmonization on specific types of technology in Europe. According to CEN, 'harmonization diminishes trade barriers, promotes safety, allows interoperability of products, systems and services, and promotes common technical understanding' (CEN, 2001). CEN comprises representatives from national and international standards-setting bodies (for example, British Standards Institute – BSI; International Standards Organization – ISO), representatives from industry (for example, European Confederation of Medical Devices Associations – EUCOMED) and consumer bodies (for example, European Association for the Co-operation of Consumer Representation in Standardisation – ANEC). The CEN Healthcare Forum (CHeF) promotes healthcare standardisation 'to ensure a high degree of patient safety and to support public health objectives, while breaking down international barriers to trade' (CEN, 2001).

Compared to pharmaceutical regulation, medical device regulation is generally considered to be less onerous for manufacturers (Kent and Faulkner, 2002). As noted in the section above on the device innovation process, safety concerns are often less pronounced in device assessment for entry to the market, because many devices have less extensive phys-iological effects than pharmaceuticals, and those that do (for example, implants) tend to have long-term physiological effects which cannot be assessed in short-term trials. Healthcare system procurement organisa-tions may be less challenging about cost-effectiveness of medical devices, since new devices often make less impact on healthcare budg-ets than new pharmaceuticals (see Cookson and Hutton, 2003).

The GHTF addresses issues relating to harmonisation of medical device legislation, risk management in medical devices, traceability of medical devices, standardising for medical devices, harmonising med-ical device nomenclature, human tissues in medical devices and drug and device compatibility. There are technical committees working in this sector to meet the requirements of the MDD. In the European Commission Directorate Health and Consumer Protection there are 'sci-entific committees' whose purpose is to provide 'high quality scientific advice for the drafting and amendment of community rules regarding consumer protection in general and consumer health in particular'.

I have described here the regulatory framework relating to the regula-tion of medical devices in Europe, the new approach to harmonisation, the role of the regulatory authorities in post-marketing surveillance and noted the development of transnational institutions for standard set-ting. It is worth emphasising that risk assessment and conformity assessment is the responsibility of medical device manufacturers together with notified bodies, overseen by the 'competent authority', which in the UK (England and Wales) is the Medicines and Healthcare products Regulatory Agency.

Comparative case studies

The world of medical devices is a socio-technological world, a world of innovation, and it is a world partly constituted by an industrial econ-omy and partly by the regulatory healthcare state. To this point in the book I have introduced the key approaches to be considered in under-standing the innovation of medical devices into healthcare systems. In the case studies that follow, the different interrelationships of the socio-technological characteristics of particular devices that engender dynam-ics of innovation and diffusion will be analysed. Taking a commitment to the comparative method, I first outline the major dynamics of the innovation pathway of each device technology, paying particular atten-tion to issues of material technology, scientific evidence, governance developments and the status of usership in relation to the technology.

A particular aim of the case studies, therefore, is to use the comparative method, taking device technologies as the key comparator (cf. Faulkner and Kent, 2001). Comparative approaches have many virtues, including the ability to identify trends, to highlight differences deserving explanation and interpretation, to point towards socio-economic dynamics underlying comparative data, to contribute to mapping fields of enquiry and to produce indicators of novel societal developments.

The five very diverse technologies exhibit a number of differences and similarities in the patterning of their social and political characteristics. More concretely, I describe the technological artefact itself; the stakeholders, including industry, regulatory agencies and users; 'evidentiality' – the scientific, surveillance-related and other evidence constructed as salient to innovation and governance; and the governance process, including state and non-state actors, legislative and informal modes, national and EU-wide. Geographically, or geopolitically, the focus is on the United Kingdom[1] and the EU because it is here that much of the formal device regulation is framed, as noted in the section above. The timescale that I focus on in the cases is notionally around the period since 1990. This is because in the UK, this marked the inauguration of the era of the new healthcare sciences ('evidence-based medicine', health technology assessment, and 'health services research') prompted partly by an increase in the budget of the NHS that was to be devoted to research and development in healthcare services as opposed to biomedicine (Faulkner, 1997).

4
Artificial Hips: The Surveillance of Success

Introduction

Recipients of artificial hips are not all as fortunate as William Jefferies, whose prosthesis, according to a BBC report, having been received in 1947 during war service in Burma, was still intact 60 years later in 2007. Contemporary artificial hip joints are generally expected to last 15 to 20 years.

The artificial hips of today developed as a high-volume healthcare device during the 1960s and 1970s and are generally regarded as one of the greatest success stories of twentieth century technological medicine (LeFanu, 2000). They are used for replacement of the hip joint mainly for people suffering pain and functional deterioration due to osteoarthritis or rheumatoid arthritis, and for the majority of implantees they provide both pain relief and improvement of locomotor function. The procedure is one of the most widely used in surgery worldwide. Hundreds of thousands of people benefit from these internally fixed mobility aids. The hip is a ball and socket joint in which the head of the thigh bone fits into and rotates in the socket of the pelvis. Most hip replacement involves replacing the femoral head of the thigh bone and the socket with artificial devices (see Figure 4.1).

Paradoxically, artificial hips have attracted an enormous degree of controversy and regulatory scrutiny over the last 20 years. In the early 1990s, like the issue of prostate cancer screening, the UK's national NHS R&D HTA programme rated hip prostheses as one of its top ten priorities. The problem was seen as a proliferation of new and often expensive designs of the technology and a parallel variation in patterns of clinical choice of models. This degree of concern was reproduced in other countries worldwide. The possible risks from human implant technologies in particular were highlighted during the 1990s by high-profile controversies (Faulkner & Kent, 2001). The total hip replacement procedure itself, aside from the technology, is very expensive and with an ageing population increasingly large numbers of potential implantees have been coming forward. Thus it appeared to the health-care policy community that here was a technology whose design, adoption and diffusion were out of control.

The healthcare products industries have been a relatively invisible actor. The orthopaedic device sector of the industry has taken advantage of the success of hip prostheses to produce a wide range of different devices aimed to serve a larger market (especially younger, fitter patients and more elderly patients). The orthopaedic device industry represents a powerful force for regulators, surgeons, healthcare providers and consumers to engage with. There is a need to understand better the development of orthopaedic hip technology itself and the routes by which different technologies reach clinical practice. Patterns of use of different types of artificial hip vary surprisingly widely between countries and regions. The devices have been subject to a great deal of assessment in national HTA organisations. Some Scandinavian countries have used registry surveillance systems since the late 1970s and early 1980s, and this tool of governance has recently been adopted in the UK. In terms of medical device regulation, in Europe all human implants such as artificial hips and breast implants have recently been reassessed for their level of risk.

The chapter provides a historical sketch of the development of the technology pointing out the trial and error culture that orthopaedic commentators have noted. Different forms of participation in the user-ship of artificial hips and clinical decision making are illustrated. A notable failure in the performance of one model of hip prosthesis in the UK is presented. I analyse the part played by regulatory agencies including NICE and procurement agencies in producing evidence-related guidance in the UK. I consider the significance of the characteristics of the device itself as a factor in shaping governance of its innovation pathway.

Epidemiology and the marketplace

Total hip replacement technology has been developed for severe degenerative joint disease, the two main conditions being osteoarthritis and rheumatoid arthritis, characterised by impairment of locomotor function and pain. Osteoarthritis is associated with advancing age while rheumatoid arthritis is more likely to occur in young adults.

Other diseases treated by the procedure include avascular necrosis, congenital dislocation, Paget's disease, ankylosing spondylitis and traumatic arthritis. Total hip replacement is generally recognised to be of great benefit in pain relief and mobility. There is evidence from clinical and health services research that implantees' quality of life is generally improved. It is most commonly used among people in their 60s and 70s, but increasing numbers of younger and older people are becoming candidates. Developments of the technology are continually introduced. Apart from younger patients where a particular issue is the expected survival of the prosthesis and its possible removal and replacement during the patient's lifetime, manufacturers also project heavier patients and very active people as other niche markets – with different implications for technology design.

Artificial hips have been implanted in the UK routinely since the mid 1960s. The proliferation of different design features and materials is spectacular. In the mid 1990s, there were over 60 different named models available in the UK. About half of these had been introduced within the previous seven to eight years. Newer models are generally more expensive. A similar number was again reported in the UK in 2003, provided by 16 companies (NAO, 2003). The Norwegian national register of artificial hip implants (see below – Governance) in the early 1990s had yielded a count of over 400 different designs and sizes of socket component and nearly 400 stem components, which was felt by the orthopaedic surgeon reporting this to be, 'from a medical point of view unreasonable' (Havelin et al., 1993). In the early 2000s, 43,000 primary (first-time) hip replacements were performed in the NHS with around 8–10,000 in the private sector (NJR/NAO, 2006).

The world annual market value for the orthopaedic implant business was estimated at around $9 billion in the late 1990s (DePuy, 1997). In the mid 2000s, one estimate of the market share for orthopaedic reconstruction overall was: Smith & Nephew eight per cent; Biomet nine per cent; DePuy (Johnson & Johnson) 19 per cent; Stryker 21 per cent; Zimmer 25 per cent; others 18 per cent (Smith & Nephew website, http://global.smith-nephew.com/master/6600.htm, 2007; figures for 2005). The market is thus dominated by six large multinational companies. For historical reasons not dwelt upon here, these companies nearly all have their headquarters in the town of Warsaw, Indiana, USA. A typical company produces a range of different implants using different materials and design concepts. Biomet, for example, in March 1999 listed 17 different trademarked femoral components and 11 socket components in its information for surgeons (Biomet, 1999).

Development of hip prosthesis technology

The material composition and design of hip prostheses is relevant to understanding the evidential science and governance of innovation of the device into the healthcare system. Risks to safety, functional performance and diversification of models arise directly from the materials and design of the technology, in combination with surgical factors and patient characteristics which shape the case-mix that surgeons deal with.

The development of orthopaedic technology has been characterised as a 'trial and error culture' among some of its own practitioners (Huiskes, 1993). There have been many examples of technological failures in the early history of the development of the device (Faulkner, 2002). The search for biocompatibility and functional performance has drawn on a wide range of materials and design concepts. In the case of hip technology, the first substantial developments can be dated to the 1950s. One single broad design concept has emerged but it cannot be said that the technology has been stabilised. Experimentation continues. The dominant concept is of a two-component device, firstly a femoral (thigh bone) strut inserted inside the femur itself, often with the addition of a fixing 'cement' and combined with a 'ball', and secondly an acetabular ('hip bone') socket component into which the ball fits and swivels (see Figure 4. 1).

The early history of the development of total hip replacement (THR) technology is shared between Europe and the US (Anderson et al., 2007).

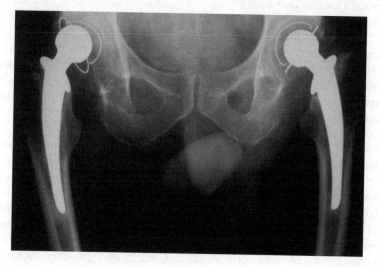

Figure 4.1 Total hip replacement in both hips

English pioneers have a strong claim to have been the inventors and developers of the first successful applications (Reynolds and Tansey, 2007), although other notable contributions were made in the US, France and Germany. The British invention and development in the field has been described as a cottage industry (Neary and Pickstone, 2007). The 1950s and 1960s were marked by a small number of hospital-based surgeons who experimented with techniques and materials, and who started to link up with academic engineers, hospital engineering workshops and engineering manufacturers. These individuals were indeed good examples of the 'heterogeneous engineer' in the sociology of technology (Law, 1987; see Chapter 2). In retrospect, the most successful heterogeneous surgeon, though not the first to pursue this goal, was Sir John Charnley. One of the most widely used prostheses still bears his name. Apart from having a workshop at his home where he produced some prototype components, Charnley also made a scientific study of biomechanical engineering and lubrication in his search for low-friction materials for the joint surfaces. At this time moulded plastics technology was developing and Charnley became aware of PTFE (polytetrafluorethylene), at the time the most slippery manufactured material known to engineering science, and otherwise known by its brand name Teflon, famous for use in cooking utensils. Setbacks followed initial success with the 'low-friction arthroplasty' but newer high-density plastics were found. By the end of the 1960s Charnley had established probably the world's leading centre for hip surgery in a former tuberculosis hospital in Wrightington, Lancashire.[1]

The range of different hip prostheses can be divided into a small number of different types and phases of innovation. In the 1970s, high failure rates of the early THRs were found. The cause was considered by many to be 'cement disease'. Although cement disease as a biological concept was and is disputed, this belief was a major stimulus in the search for alternative solutions. Various cement-free methods have been developed which can be summarised as, firstly: press-fit methods, in which fixation is sought by closeness of fit between prosthesis and bone; secondly, porous-coated, in which surfaces are given a microporous coating in the form of mesh or beads to encourage ingrowth of bone and, thirdly, hydroxyapatite- (HA-) coated, which is similar to porous coating but the surfaces are coated with a biologically active calcium phosphate ceramic. In 'hybrid' models, a cemented stem is combined with an uncemented cup, which may retain the relatively good performance of cemented stems but substitutes possibly superior cement-free cups; this allows immediate weight-bearing and may be seen clinically as suitable for older patients unable to use crutches. The issue of hybrid models and the practice of surgeons 'mixing and matching' their own choice of components has come to the attention of the regulatory authorities. This is discussed below. The latest significant development is the fully modular type of prosthesis, in which a range of sizes of separate subcomponents of the total prosthesis are made available as a 'hip system'.

The main materials used in contemporary hip implants are metals, plastics and ceramics. The 'same' model is often produced by manufacturers in different metals and coatings. The bearing surface materials of the femoral head and socket component also vary widely. The arrival of superalloys and composite materials has almost eliminated mechanical breakage in normal usage of the artificial hip. The stronger, new materials appear to have brought with them their own problems, and these may appear only two or three years after implantation. Small changes may have large consequences. This issue is explored below in the controversial case of the 'Capital' hip technology.

The medical device industry promotes the newer materials and design concepts. For example Eucomed, the European medical device industry trade association, describes the benefits of porous-coated hips as follows:

> One ... advancement is the use of porous hip implants. As technology has advanced, the use of cemented implants has shifted, with a large percentage of orthopaedic surgeons now using porous hip implants.
>
> (Eucomed, 2007a)

Eucomed claims a range of benefits for this type of technology including better fit, long-term stability via bone growing into the implant, reduced operating time and enablement of minimally invasive surgical techniques (Eucomed, op. cit.). The equivocal scientific evidence about this and the other main types of novel fixation technology for the hip is discussed in the section below on science.[2]

Innovating orthopaedic surgeons, bioengineering research laboratories and manufacturers often form strategic alliances to bring new designs to the stage of clinical experimentation (see Anderson et al., 2007: Chapter 4). Technological innovation in the artificial hip extends to research in stem cells and tissue engineering, the topic of the fifth case study in this book. For example, one EU funded international project is examining the use of cord blood stem cells in repairing bone defects and fractures (Anon, 2007). The possibility of a prosthetic technology carrying live human cells has been the subject of debate among policymakers in the EU debating the regulation of cell-based technologies at the boundary of pharmaceuticals, tissues and medical devices. This is discussed in the case study of tissue engineered technology in Chapter 8.

I now discuss the material and social forces shaping the usership of hip prostheses and consider the question of how users might shape technological innovation and the variable patterns of availability of the device in the healthcare system.

Usership and practice

The usership of artificial hips is split between surgeons and patients. Usership of artificial hips should be considered in several dimensions. Most obviously, surgeon users are presented with a commercial marketplace of different models. The social and organisational structuring of the orthopaedic profession, the national and local policies of healthcare purchasing and providers, the marketing policies of manufacturers and hospital policies about clinical trials of new models of the device, mean that the user is set at a distance from issues of availability and choice. Various other constituencies have an interest in data on performance of the technology once implanted: the individual consultant, surgical team, hospital or treatment centre and broader regional or national authorities.

Because hip replacement is an iconic procedure in healthcare in the UK, frequently the subject of parliamentary comment because of the numbers of patients 'waiting to have their hip done', it is often the subject of reports in the broadcast media. This is one of the reasons for the high level of exposure of the orthopaedic profession to government and public inquiries over the last 15 years. From a consumerist perspective, proliferation of models can be regarded as offering 'more choice' to the consumer. Patients' access to information about their implants has often been limited, however. Hip implantees do not in general have a collective identity. Citizens have limited resources to question widely held beliefs that hip replacement offers an improved quality of life and assumptions that clinicians, manufacturers and regulators are acting in their best interest. It is certain that most implantees have not had detailed information about the design and material composition of their artificial hips.

In the early 1990s, concern about the surgical procedure of hip replacement inflamed the mass media imagination (for example, *The Guardian*, 'Shooting at the Hip', 23 February 1993 – 'Shoddy material and inept surgeons mean that up to 30 per cent of hip replacements have to be redone'), and a television programme focused upon 'The High Price Of Hips' (BBC2, 1993). Concern was also expressed by leading spokesmen (yes, men) within the orthopaedic profession itself, suggesting that there were potentially risky trends in hip implantation developing (Murray et al., 1995; Bulstrode et al., 1993). This was described derogatorily as a trend toward 'designer hips'.

End users: implantees

The population of hip recipients is diverse, with somewhat more females than males, but lacking collective identity. There are no organised groups for hip implantees, though some internet-based 'self-help' networks are emerging.

It is significant that in the 1990s in the UK the high-profile independent general consumer organisation, the Consumers Association, reported on hip implants with an account that highlighted issues of the 'untested' status of many models as well as the variability in surgeons' performance (*Health Which?*, 1997; see Figure 4.2).

Usership of artificial hips should also be defined to include the embodied experience of patients. While there is a great deal of evidence about the outcome of total hip replacement produced by orthopaedic surgeons using established clinical monitoring tools (measuring gait, pain and so on), there is less that employs qualitative methods to assess patients' experiences and very little indeed that attempts to present the patient's experience of the prosthesis itself. Interestingly, the few published qualitative studies that have been produced have come largely from nursing specialists. The reported return-to-home experience of hip recipients is, as one would expect, focused mainly on 'normal' lifestyle. One qualitative study from Japan interviewed patients suffering osteoarthritis before and after the surgical procedure. The study revealed some distress about body image in patients following the implantation: 'The ... participants gradually became used to life with the prosthesis so that the feelings of strangeness about the prosthesis started to wear off' (Fujita et al., 2006). There is little academic research that sheds further light on people's bodily experience of hip implants and the meanings with which the devices are construed, unless problems occur. It is generally assumed that concern about the functionality of the devices is the overriding frame of reference for implantees. Anecdotally, the media-fuelled image of the 'bionic man/woman' is often drawn upon by patients. Some research under way at the time of writing should add significantly to our understanding here (Hoeyer, 2007).

In the early 1990s, healthcare and clinical scientists began to see a need for 'patient-based outcome measures' and 'Quality of life' measures

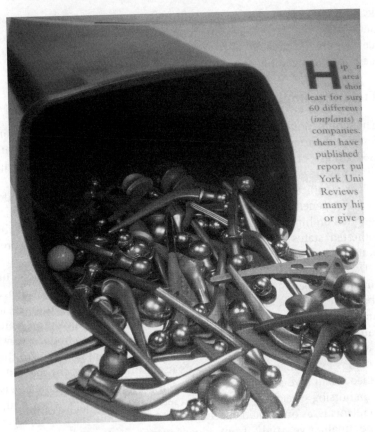

Within the figure image, partial text is visible:

> H ip r
> area
> shor
> least for surg
> 60 different i
> (*implants*) a
> companies.
> them have
> published
> report pul
> York Uni
> Reviews
> many hip
> or give p

Figure 4.2 Artificial hip controversy in the public sphere

specific to particular clinical interventions. For example, a medical sociol-ogist and orthopaedic surgeons collaborated to develop a hip-specific quality of life tool (Dawson et al., 1996). The questionnaire assesses pain and activities such as washing, using transport, dressing, walking and interference with work and sleep. In general, studies using such measure-ment tools report very favourable quality of life experiences for hip implantees.

Such tools have become standardised as Patient Reported Outcome Measurement (PROMs). In a development illustrating the extension of monitoring activity, the UK's National Joint Registry (NJR), discussed further below, convened a PROM studies group in 2004. Its stated purposes are: To demonstrate patient benefit from total hip/total knee replacement; and to undertake 'Surveillance: using outcomes data to improve quality standards for: Components; Surgical technique; and Surgical/hospital performance'; also to 'listen to patients' and to contribute to internal audit within hospitals (NJR Centre, 2005).

Among patients, clearly the end-user experience and understanding of artificial hips is mediated by the beliefs and practices of surgeons, and the mass media have intervened on some issues. The fact of the discreteness of the material technology and its invisibility once implanted, and the fact that end-users do not interact with it, are clearly salient to their individual and societal meanings. Their overriding significance lies in their performance as artificial replacements for bodily function and sensation. The wide variety of materials and designs that are available is all the more striking set in this context of user functionality.

Surgeon-consumers

The involvement of orthopaedic surgeons in design and development continues, although the extent and nature of the participation is difficult to estimate. Some surgeons are also commercial entrepreneurs. A small interview study of orthopaedic surgeons conducted in the mid 1990s in connection with one of the UK HTA systematic reviews showed the way in which surgeons might be enrolled into using a particular device:

> [T]he Müller ... they do run courses in Switzerland to which they partially reimburse you, and it's a very well run course – scientific, well documented ... I don't go every year but they are there ... and they also pay for one middle grade (i.e. trainee) to go.
>
> (Donovan, 1997)

For some models of prosthesis the degree of involvement may be very great. All six surgeons in this small study reported at least some contact with manufacturers. Some were involved in developing modifications to the equipment required to perform the procedure, and one reported a high level of involvement in developing the implant itself:

> I have a lot of contact with them ... we have regular development meetings ... and discuss advancement and modifications ... Professor XX invented the X hip and the successor, so in fact we ... don't quite *tell* them what to do but ... they tend to take our advice ... they do follow our, er, instructions.
>
> (Donovan,1997)

Manufacturers, of course, themselves attempt to exercise direct influence on surgeons' choice of prosthesis through sales staff and marketing strategies:

> Int: Is there much pressure to change to different implants?
>
> Surgeon 3: No, no. Well they'll ... when you are appointed they come and try to get you but once you are established they ... don't tend to push it too much ... they do come and show their wares.
>
> Surgeon 4: You get the manufacturers coming in ... once a month they come with these fancy boxes of tricks and the open them up over the floor of the fracture clinic ... and somebody like me really has no idea whether they're talking rubbish or talking sense ... I think it's probably true of a great many of my colleagues in this country, er, the new model looks better like the new model car looks better. But it can go wrong ... You've got to be awfully careful.
>
> (Donovan, 1997 op. cit.)

So the majority of surgeons engage with manufacturers as specialist consumers of a complex array of a range of models and brands.

Technological practice patterns

The observation of patterns of variation in healthcare delivery has been one of the springboards for the upsurge in Health Services Research generally (Wennberg and Gittelsohn, 1982; and famously Wennberg et al., 1987). Patterns of variation of use of different hip technologies became apparent both in the UK and between different national healthcare systems during the 1990s. At this time no breakdown of numbers of people registered as receiving different types of implant was available in the UK as a whole (Murray et al., 1995). A survey published in 1993 (Newman, 1993) showed that 70 per cent of orthopaedic centres in the UK used both the more conventional 'cemented' and less conventional 'uncemented' modes of fixation to some extent. In the UK the most common prosthesis (the 'Charnley' cemented model) was used in between 40 per cent and 50 per cent of primary hip replacements in the UK. Patterns of different models of hip prostheses suggest that relatively stable, shared institutional practices exist within healthcare provider organisations and associated orthopaedic professional networks.

In spite of the internationally shared nature of many hospital surgical procedures, there were also variations between countries. One of the

Table 4.1 Range of artificial hip components used in England and Wales.

Year	Reported number of different femoral components	Reported number of different acetabular components	Number of combinations	% 'mixed and matched'
2004	101	88	574	25%
2005	129	110	ca. 790	25%
2006	176	155	776	22%

Source: Data from National Joint Registry annual reports, years 2004 to 2006, compiled by the author.

most conspicuous examples was that in Finland over 50 per cent of hips were non-cemented while in neighbouring Sweden and Norway the percentages were 4 per cent and 15 per cent respectively (Havelin et al., 1993), strongly suggesting the influence of non-clinical forces shaping orthopaedic practice. There is evidence of similar patterns of differences in the early 2000s.

Variation in patterns of practice has continued in the mid 2000s. As shown in Table 4.1, the range of different types of model of components appears to be increasing, although this is partly an artefact caused by the gradual increase in numbers of hospitals providing data to the NJR.

In 2004 most reported procedures used cement, but since then there has been a trend towards more cementless procedures. Somewhat older than average patients received cemented prostheses and non-cemented models were used in a higher proportion of younger patients.

An important and controversial practice among surgeons has been to combine a femoral component (incorporating a metallic or ceramic modular head) from one manufacturer with an acetabular component (incorporating a plastic bearing surface) from another. The practice is known as 'Mixing and Matching' or sometimes cross-breeding. As seen in the Table 4.1, this practice of professional discretion is very common, with around one quarter of replacements taking this form in the UK. The practice has been controversial among manufacturers and among regulatory agencies. This is discussed below in the section on governance.

In summary, the type of hip replacement a patient receives depends on which country and which region they have the operation in, and upon local orthopaedic technology purchasing policy, clinical beliefs and surgical socialisation structures. A key point in this discussion has been the incremental innovation in the technology. The issue of small variations to apparently established designs was highlighted in the UK in the late 1990s by apparent problems with one particular model of hip. This incident was significant for the development of the healthcare science and governance of artificial hips and I discuss this case in the following section.

A controversy and an enquiry

The 'Capital' artificial hip

In the case of artificial hips, an incident with the 'Capital' Hip System was a high profile instance of apparent failure of a hip prosthesis in the UK during the 1990s. The Capital hip was introduced, to the UK market only, in 1991 by the healthcare division of the multi-sector American-owned manufacturing company 3M. It was a relatively cheap variant of the industry-standard 'Charnley' prosthesis, and was available in a single-piece stainless steel version and a modular titanium alloy version. They were implanted into about 4700 patients in the UK up to 1997.

In 1998 the government regulatory body, the MDA, issued a notice alerting the healthcare providers to apparent failures of the technology. 3M Healthcare, while not admitting that the device was defective, nor admitting formal liability, were to fund a process of recall and re-operation (undertaken via the private sector healthcare provider BUPA). The company stated that the device had been withdrawn from the market for commercial reasons. The implant had been the subject of an initial clinical report suggesting problems with the device from one orthopaedic surgical centre (Nottingham), which was presented at the annual conference of the British Orthopaedic Association (BOA) of 1995. The paper, typical of the reports of orthopaedic device performance at the time, having small numbers of patients/hips and a short length of surveillance of clinical results, was published later by the Journal of Bone and Joint Surgery (Massoud et al., 1997). The report suggested that 26 per cent of the 89 implanted devices had failed due to femoral loosening at an average of 26 months. Unusually, and controversially for many of those attending, the company had been granted a 'right of reply' to the evidence presented by the surgeons. A later informal account of this exchange (in e-discussion list arthroplasty@mailbase.ac.uk) concluded that the company's position was essentially that the surgeons in question had been using an inappropriate technique.

The Capital was of concern within some parts of the orthopaedic profession. Subsequently further results have been published from other centres in the UK suggesting that failure was widespread (Pandit et al., 2000). However, such 'scientific' research reports, based as they are upon a single series of patients operated upon by a single group of surgeons in a single surgical centre, are notoriously regarded as statistically weak due to confounding factors (e.g. surgical technique, severity of patients' conditions or activity levels). Thus the strength of the 'evidence' for the failure of the prosthesis was not as robust as might be assumed, especially on the basis of the first one or two reports.

To give an idea of the complexity of the technology, it is worth illustrating the extremely fine-grained variation of material and components in this type of device:

> The system offered two geometrically identical types of stem ... a single-unit head and neck made of stainless steel, and the Capital which was a modular system with a titanium-alloy stem and a choice of heads. The stem was either of standard geometry which was approximately the same as the Charnley roundback 40, or of flanged which differed from the Charnley in that it was wider and more conical, without shouldering. Both had a shot-blasted, rough-surface finish.
>
> (McGrath et al., 2001)

These authors suggested that the stainless steel model 'should be considered as a different prosthesis' (op. cit.). Further published reports appeared to confirm that there were problems with the technology (including Davies et al., 1999; Pandit et al., 2000), though this has also been attributed to the type of cement used (Roy et al., 2002). Published calls from within the profession for improvement to governance arrangements via surveillance were increasing (for example, Pandit et al., 2000).

There was no consensus within the orthopaedic profession or between orthopaedic surgeons, the manufacturer and the regulatory authority regarding the cause of the failure. The recall sparked an investigation instigated by the UK Department of Health. This included senior members of the British Orthopaedic Association, members of the MDA and manufacturer 3M representatives. The investigation was based at the Royal College of Surgeons (RCS). The RCS report was unable to identify unequivocally the technical cause of the failure. Three years after the initial hazard notice, this investigation concluded that design modifications should be evaluated fully by the collection of data on performance post-marketing or through controlled trials; that an orthopaedic joint registry be established to assist with post-marketing surveillance and that better records be kept by surgeons carrying out hip replacements. Inadequacies in the quality of post-marketing information and poor record keeping in healthcare institutions were highlighted.

The Capital incident received considerable adverse mass media press coverage, and was commented upon in the British Parliament. One UK member of Parliament was reported to have said that, compared to orthopaedic device design and manufacturing, 'quality control is better on a lawnmower'! The incident added fuel to the growing perceived need for improved regulation. This is discussed further in the section below on governance.

Science

Healthcare science

During the late 1980s and early 1990s, at the time when the evidence-based movements were starting to gather momentum, some members of the orthopaedic profession were starting to question the methods by which their surgical practices and results should be evaluated. Practical problems are acknowledged with applying the lengthy Randomised Control Trial (RCT) approach in the case of a technology where there is a high level of innovation (Laupacis et al., 1989). The long periods of follow-up required if performance is measured by the need for a revision prosthesis was also criticised, as was the use of conventional clinical scores of pain, walking function and so on. These were criticised for their inability to distinguish between the effects of the different components of the prosthesis. Thus some surgeons advocated the development of predictive measurement techniques such as migration analysis, using computer-assisted analysis of radiological measurement of short-term movement of the implanted prosthesis *in situ*. However, it appeared in time that the correlation was poor between results of this type of imaging analysis with clinical or patient-derived evaluation of the performance of the technology.

Members of the orthopaedic profession were also becoming concerned about the proliferation of prostheses. In a high profile article deliberately titled to evoke the consumerisation of the orthopaedic marketplace, leading surgeons from Oxford in the UK asked 'Which primary total hip replacement?' (Murray et al., 1995). They criticised the lack of scientific evidence especially about newer more expensive implants, and made one of the first significant recommendations that surgeons should prefer implants with 'good results in published peer-reviewed long-term clinical trials'. The authors, as noted above, had already published a critique of 'designer hips' in an editorial in the *British Medical Journal* (Bulstrode et al., 1993). New implants should be subject to 'clinical testing as well as laboratory wear testing' before release. It was noted that the then recent introduction of the CE mark through the European Union device Directive was an important opportunity to 'rationalise the implant market in Europe' (Murray et al., 1995).

The issue of the effectiveness of hip prostheses was given high priority on the Department of Health policy and R&D agendas. The NHS Centre for Reviews and Dissemination, key intermediary in the NHS strategy for a knowledge-based health service, had commissioned the first National Health Service mandated review of evidence of artificial hip effectiveness (NHS CRD, 1997) against the background of concern (Wearne and Jones, 1993).

Subsequently, like the PSA test for prostate cancer, it was made one of the highest priorities for systematic review of evidence in the initial work of the UK national HTA programme. The HTA studies focused on the comparative effectiveness and cost-effectiveness of different hip prostheses (Faulkner et al., 1998; Fitzpatrick et al., 1998). The reports reviewed hundreds of mainly single series studies internationally, although attempts were made at meta-analysis (Fitzpatrick et al.) and maximising the evidence from comparative studies (Faulkner et al.). There was no published evidence about the 3M Capital prosthesis at the time so neither review included reference to it. The HTA studies recommended the development of patient-oriented evaluation of the technology: 'Further inclusion of patient-derived quality-of-life measures in studies of hip prosthesis performance is essential, as clinical hip-scoring systems do not take the patient's views into account when assessing outcomes' (Faulkner et al., op. cit.). Both reports recommended that a registry system, similar to those already established in some Scandinavian countries, should be considered for the UK.

It is interesting that most HTA scientific attention has focused upon the issue of alternative models and materials of hip implant. This emphasis, or bias, was reflected also in the way in which the healthcare policy communities have framed the problems of artificial hips. This is discussed in the next section. This focus downplays other variables that influence the performance of the hip replacement procedure, notably the skill of the surgeon and the 'approach' i.e. the surgical route by which the procedure is undertaken. The number of studies assessing these factors, compared to the technology of the prosthesis, has been very small indeed. While it is not discussed in detail here, Neary (2007) has described how design of prosthesis and different surgical approaches have been interdependent. More recently, the techniques of minimally invasive surgery have been introduced into hip replacement procedures, and this also is having an effect on design and the patterns of use of different materials and designs (Eucomed, 2007a).

Policy and governance

The regulatory environment of hip prostheses in the UK was relatively unrestrictive during the 1980s and early 1990s. A surveillance scheme based on a 'recommended list', a limited number of models agreed to be acceptable, had been agreed between the government and the orthopaedic profession in 1981 (Sweetnam, 1981), but it was not implemented. Unlike some other implants, there was no national registry of clinical implant information, voluntary or otherwise, although one regional health authority area (Trent) established a monitoring system of this type in 1990. Although orthopaedic departments and centres generally were taken to record the prostheses implanted in their own patients, there was no co-ordination of these data. As the issue began to climb the healthcare policy agenda, this situation was increasingly contrasted with the Scandinavian countries, which had established registries – in Sweden in 1979, Finland in 1980 and in Norway in 1987. Thus at this time only pre-clinical technological product testing had been mandatory, under 'good manufacturing practice' regulations, which called for technological bench tests and biocompatibility assessments.

Total hip prostheses became a site for increasing attempts at regulatory activity in various forms in the UK during the 1990s. It is clear in this technology that processes of innovation outpace the development of regulatory controls. The interests of manufacturers, and the philosophy of a free market in Europe, promote pressures for harmonisation of technical standards. Countries vary in their arrangements for surveillance of implanted devices. From an HTA perspective the published clinical studies in orthopaedic journals have been of limited usefulness for evaluation of effectiveness of prostheses because numbers are generally small, follow-up periods relatively short and opportunities for pooling data limited (Faulkner et al., 1998).

Innovation and proliferation: Designer hips

A measure of the very high profile that artificial hips issues achieved within the surgical profession generally, is that the 1996 Hunterian lecture, the annual showpiece lecture for the Royal College of Surgeons, was devoted to considering the 'way forward' for this technology (Bulstrode, 1996). The performance of the newer non-cemented models has been controversial within the orthopaedic profession. One surgical commentator has described the effects of the new materials as 'a torrent of particles into our joints, producing a devastation far exceeding simple prosthetic failure or fragmentation of parts' (Booth, 1994). This may be an exaggerated account, but does point to the continual emergence of new potential problems (cf. Styles et al., 1998). Thus there is little doubt that the clinical effects of the new combinations of materials have raised regulatory concerns about the safety of the technologies and their evaluation.

As the Capital incident showed, small variations in design could have major consequences. An editorial in the primary academic journal of orthopaedic surgery commented that the Capital:

> has led both the public and orthopaedic surgeons to question the effectiveness of existing controls in the UK which govern the introduction of new prostheses for joint replacement ... Such a 'look-alike' prosthesis may be difficult to identify and test ... It is therefore important that orthopaedic surgeons involve themselves in this process ... to retain the confidence and support of the public.
>
> (Grigoris and Hamblen, 1998)

It was notable that an immediate consequence of the Capital incident was the production of British Orthopaedic Association guidance which included a new reference to the possible risk arising from small variations to existing designs (BOA, 1999). Thus orthopaedic surgery was moving towards increased self-regulation and participation in governance processes.

The general surgical profession has also involved itself in the evaluation of hip implant procedures in the NHS. The RCS of England published a National Total Hip Replacement Outcomes Study in 2000. The MDA acted on a suggestion made by the British Hip Society (BHS – a subgroup of the British Orthopaedic Association) in 2002 that a group of experienced orthopaedic surgeons should be available to advise on 'Adverse Incidents' that are reported to them. The committee is known as the Orthopaedic Advisory Committee and involves MDA (MHRA), the president of the BOA and representatives from the BHS. This is another example of the orthopaedic community actively seeking representation of their interests in the regulatory arena.

The UK Department of Health and orthopaedic surgeons' professional association debated the value of registries. Approval was given to the proposal to set up a joint registry following the recommendations of the investigation into the performance of the 3M Capital hip system by the RCS (RCS, 2001). The Capital hip incident investigators produced the following conclusion, pointing to problems with implementation of EU device regulations:

> Although the new regulations are intended to ensure that new prostheses undergo more rigorous evaluation prior to their introduction, they cannot be relied upon to prevent a hip prosthesis with poor performance similar to the modular flanged Capital hip coming to the market in the future. This lack of confidence in the regulations arises, in part, because of the potential for differing interpretations of the regulations in Europe.
>
> (RCS, 2001, p. 82)

The reference here is to the device Directives which allow some flexibility in certifying authorities' interpretation of what constitutes adequate evidence of safety in dossiers presented in support of marketing authorisation decisions. The principle of 'proportionality' means that small variations to an existing design were likely to require a lesser rigour and depth of supporting data. In the UK, the MHRA requires manufacturers and trusts to report all incidents of prosthetic failure and loosening and circumstances where the reason for revision surgery is unclear. This is part of their responsibility as the 'competent authority' under the EU medical device directives' vigilance system. However, the reporting rate is generally taken to be not as high as the regulator would expect.

Guidance to healthcare providers

Since the publication of the two UK HTA systematic reviews in 1998 (Faulkner et al.; Fitzpatrick et al., 1998), there have been further developments in regulatory policy for artificial hips. These reviews contributed directly and explicitly to the knowledge on which NICE's guidance to the health service was based, issued first in March 2000. The primary guidance is that 'the best prostheses demonstrate a revision rate (the rate at which they need to be replaced) of 10 per cent or less at 10 years. This should be regarded as the current benchmark in the selection of prostheses for primary Total Hip Replacement' (NICE, 2000a). This guidance was in line with the principle introduced in 1998 that revision of primary hip replacement due to aseptic loosening within 10 years of implantation should be reportable to the MDA (MDA, 1998). NICE also specified evidential requirements for the criteria for demonstrating adequate performance of a prosthesis. These included: 10 or more years follow-up from multi-centre studies; randomised controlled trials or adequately sized, well-conducted observational studies with consecutive patients from unbiased populations. However, in spite of the central importance of the establishment of the 10-10 (ten-year/ten percent) performance criterion, NICE later added what arguably was an easing of this rule, namely that it was 'reasonable to consider' prostheses with at least three years of follow-up if performance was 'consistent with' the 10-10 benchmark.[3]

Surveillance and investigation

The British government has also concerned itself directly with artificial hips. The National Audit Office (NAO), the financial 'watchdog' of the British government, produced a wide-ranging report on many aspects of hip replacement in the NHS (NAO, 2000), followed by an update (NAO, 2003). These reports note some progress but continuing weaknesses in regard to systems of surveillance of implanted hips, NHS Trust policies for introduction of new prostheses, variations in performance across the NHS, concerns about the use of incentives by manufacturers, surgical training and expertise, under-reporting of adverse incidents and compliance with NICE guidance. The 2003 report is critical of the ten per cent of orthopaedic surgeons 'who have no adequate evidence of effectiveness for the prostheses they use'. The NAO shows concern that incentives are offered by prosthesis manufacturers to NHS Trusts and to consultants to use new versions (60 out of 650 had accepted incentives, mainly free overseas travel to training events). Such incentives to trusts 'may unduly influence their purchasing decisions'. In 2003 it was also found that fewer NHS trusts had policies for the introduction of new prostheses than in 1999. Recommendations for improvement were made (NAO, 2003).

Concerns in the British Parliament persist. In 2004 the Public Accounts Committee assessed the issue and MPs said controls were needed on the use of new types of artificial hip, which had little or no track record of effectiveness (BBC, 2004). Their investigation found that 40 per cent of trusts had been offered incentives by manufacturers to switch to new models. The NHS Purchasing and Supply Agency (PASA) was urged to issue a list of prostheses that meet the published standards.

Finally, it should be noted that there had been a variety of calls from various quarters, increasingly strong since the mid-1990s, for the introduction of a 'registry' system in the UK for the recording of all hip (and knee) replacements. Surgeons' opinion on this had begun to shift. The Capital controversy certainly added fuel to the debate about this. The Department of Health issued a formal consultation document on the registry proposal (Department of Health, 2000) and a system, after a great deal of debate and negotiation between the stakeholders involved, was announced in July 2001 and launched in April 2003 (reported in National Audit Office, 2003). It is a voluntary system, funded by a volume-dependent levy on NHS Trusts.

Technology adoption policy

Regulatory attention to hip devices has also been marshalled around the purchasing process for the NHS in the UK. The surveillance activity here is part of the more general government-promoted steerage toward evidence-based purchasing. As noted in the introductory chapter on governance in this book, the strategic *rapprochement* of scientific evidence-production and purchasing policy is one of the most significant innovations in regulatory policy in the last decade. The issue of control over the purchasing of orthopaedic technology has been such that the NHS' centralised purchasing policy agency now hosts a specific Orthopaedic Data Evaluation Panel (ODEP). NHS PASA requested the industry to submit evidence for prostheses claimed to meet NICE's 10-year benchmark. ODEP's function is to provide an independent assessment of these clinical data and of compliance with the benchmarks. According to the criteria agreed for ODEP and NHS PASA, 28 per cent of the stems and 37 per cent of the sockets entered into the National Joint Registry met the NICE 10-year benchmark in 2006. However, the ODEP report could only refer to brands that were introduced more than 10 years previously and a considerable number of brands have been introduced since. Evaluations of evidence submitted by industry are graded by years of available data and quality of the data, and a classification is awarded. Thus, for example, the Charnley Standard Cup first used in 1962 and produced by DePuy has the highest possible rating, and the Charnley Modular cemented stem, first used in 1988 and produced by the same company, has a medium classification with a note that the data supplied lacks survivorship analysis (NHS Supply Chain, 2006). Other typical criticisms of datasets were that studies were based in only a single-centre and that numbers of patients in studied cohorts were small. Products meeting the ten year benchmark in 2006 were: 69 per cent of cemented stems, 70.6 per cent cementless stems, 42.6 per cent of cemented cups and just 4.8 per cent of cementless cups (NJR, 2007).

In the light of the institutionalisation of both the 10-year and 3-year evidential benchmarks by NICE and the use of the grading and classification system by the purchasing authority's panel, it is clear that controversial issues remain for the orthopaedic community, the manufacturers and the evaluators and regulators about what benchmark to use, the scientific criteria with which to demonstrate the validity of claims of device performance and the implementation of these regulatory assessment schemes.

Standards and European regulation

The manufacture of orthopaedic implants is covered by a large number of national (for example, BSI) and international (ISO) technical standards. Coverage includes material composition and mechanical testing. A number of harmonised standards in the European Union have been produced.[4] Draft standards are circulated 'for public inquiry' to EU members (Paul, 1997). Standards generally apply to the material used in the production process rather than the finished product. Some features have proved impossible to subject to specific standards because of their variety. This applies, for example, to the modular head (ball) of femoral components (Paul, 1997).

From July 1998, following the EU device directives, clinical investigations were required under certain conditions by the MDA, in order for a CE mark to be given. These investigations are required for reasons including: where there is a 'completely new concept of device ... where components, features and/or methods of action are previously unknown'; in the case of 'modification of an existing device in such a way that it contains a novel feature'; or where existing materials are used in a new location in the human body. This system thus draws a distinction between devices that are in some sense novel and those which can be shown to have an equivalent or near-equivalent already on the market, like the Capital. The principle was thus one of 'substantial equivalence' relying on evidence that the product is technically similar to an existing device on the market and on adequate 'clinical evidence' for the *type* of product (Gelijns, 1990). Similarly, the UK's MDA in the 1990s produced guidance for manufacturers carrying out clinical investigations in the UK, including stipulations regarding study design, sample size calculation and statistical analysis (MDA, 1998).

Under its post-marketing surveillance responsibility, the MDA produced a small number of 'hazard notices' and 'safety notices' following failures of specific prosthesis components. Total hip implants were originally a Class IIb (or Class III if bioactively coated) device under the EU medical device regulatory system. Under the vigilance system, CE-marked joint replacement implants became subject to an enhanced requirement for reporting of adverse incidents by manufacturers to the MDA. Any failure of an implant attributable to premature deterioration or malfunction became reportable. This included the most common cause of implant failure, 'aseptic loosening'. Review of the clinical research reporting the performance of hip implants at the time showed that the attribution of responsibility for failure was often contentious. The cause of failure of hip implants in younger, more active people is especially likely to be contested (Faulkner et al., 1998). This implies that individual clinical assessment and local circumstances are paramount in determining whether a report is actually made following revision operations.

Artificial hips were not seen as a public health policy issue at European level before the Capital incident. There has been no end-user consumer campaign, unlike on the safety issues of breast implants (Kent, 2003). However, following the Capital incident, the regulatory authorities of two of the EU member states, UK and France, decided that the risk rating of orthopaedic and other implant technologies within the EU regime was too low. These two countries began a campaign to change the classification, a process requiring the drafting of a new directive. The campaign was eventually successful. Industry representatives tried to delay the reclassification process. Industry association Eucomed argued against the reclassification, alleging that there was no scientific justification for it and that it would bring a longer and more costly route to compliance (Maxwell, 2003).

The influence of the UK regulator's reaction to the Capital incident can clearly be seen in the reclassifying directive, which referred to 'at first sight ... minor post-marketing changes to the design of previously trouble-free replacements can lead to serious problems' (European Commission, 2005).

The new Directive stated that

> in order to achieve the optimal level of safety and health protection and to reduce the design related problems to the lowest level, the design dossier of hip, knee and shoulder replacements, including the clinical data used by the manufacturer ... should be inspected 'in detail' by the notified body under the full quality assurance system.
>
> (European Commission, 2005)

UK device regulation

The MHRA has considered the question of 'mix and match' orthopaedic implants. As noted above this is a very common practice. There has been a controversial debate on this issue between regulators, manufacturers and orthopaedic surgeons. Around 2004–5 MHRA drafted a Medical Device Alert advising clinicians against the practice of mixing and matching hip replacement implants and reminding them of the need to follow manufacturers instructions. The majority of manufacturers supported the publication but the BHS advised MHRA that they were totally opposed to it as they did not consider that there was sufficient evidence to indicate that the practice was unsafe. Representatives from MHRA, BHS (a subgroup of BOA), British Orthopaedic Association, ABHI and the Defence Unions met. As a result the industry agreed to explore the possibility of amending their instructions to allow the practice of mixing and matching to appropriate standards. In fact, there continued to be a 'low' level of reports of failure associated with this practice (CSD minutes, 2004).

In 2005 NICE reviewed their guidance on hip prostheses. Consultees in the process represented manufacturers, the NJR, the ODEP and professionals, the NICE secretariat and the Chair of its appraisal committee. It was concluded that there were no new comparative data, thus review of the guidance was deferred. A further notable development in the UK is closer working that has been designed between NICE and the NHS PASA (NICE, 2000b), producing greater interlocking of regulatory controls. NICE has approved NHS PASA's data related to benchmarking and the establishment of the ODEP, discussed above. NICE states that, with the continued support of the British Orthopaedic Association, BHS and ABHI, both PASA and the NJR can continue to play vital roles in developing valuable databases on the hip performance. Thus here we see the importance of an emerging collaborative style of regulatory institution-building and surveillance of artificial hip technology, between the range of regulatory actors.

In summary, there is a diversification of regulatory agencies taking different approaches to the gatekeeping of artificial hip innovation into the healthcare system. A triumvirate of constituencies has evolved, participating in surveillance and control of hip prosthesis technology and clinical usership. There has been a tightening of links between the evidence-based healthcare regulator NICE and the national purchasing authority which is of particular significance. HTA analyses suggest that significant improvements are required in the technology in order to improve on the cost-effectiveness of the relatively long-established cemented models. However, it is notable that cost-effectiveness is not included in the ODEP evidence-based purchasing agency's data.

Having focused on effectiveness and cost-effectiveness during the 1990s in the UK, the Capital incident came from outside the effectiveness-focused evaluation for hips. 'Lack of evidence' and methodological issues were in themselves construed as a regulatory issue, regardless of whether safety or effectiveness was the main criterion. The registry surveillance system institutionalises a methodology which combines the ability to capture safety as well as effectiveness-relevant data. At the same time the development of the data evaluation group in the central purchasing agency embeds principles of evidentiality at the centre of the adoption process. However, these developments have been criticised from a public health perspective as weak in their requirements of data from manufacturers (van der Meulen, 2005).

Dynamics of artificial hip innovation and governance

The orthopaedic community practising joint replacement underwent its own legitimation crisis during the 1990s, in a process linked to the emergence of the evidence-based healthcare policymaking movement. The overriding aim of healthcare policymakers' governance of artificial hips has been to rationalise and contain diffusion of the range of the technology. In the UK during the 1990s evidence was marshalled especially within the HTA frame. This emphasis may have produced a governance environment in which concerns about *safety* as raised by the Capital incident were all the more disruptive. The safety of the device had not been a major driving force in informing governance activity. Latterly, both pre-marketing testing and post-marketing surveillance have been enhanced, firstly through the reclassification under EU law and secondly in the UK with the establishment of the NJR.

The power of industry and the surgical professions and their relationship to each other are the key social relations in the shaping of the innovation pathway of artificial hips, and this has been counteracted – with some success – by an evidentiality focused upon clinical and health system cost criteria, orchestrated by centralised and co-ordinated national government and regulatory agencies. Commentators in the orthopaedic profession globally continue to criticise the apparent dependency of the profession upon industry (Sarmiento, 2003).

There has been no governance-related movement to create an 'informed patient' in the case of artificial hip. Although surgeons and epidemiologists deploy various techniques to codify, image and analyse the performance of the technology, the uncertainty of interpretation does not present the arthritic citizen with the same sort of life-chance dilemmas as some monitoring or testing technologies. Artificial hips are part of professional projects of socialisation, apprenticeship, knowledge-production and defined worlds of clinical practice in a way that technologies whose clinical ownership is diversified and more widely dispersed are not. Thus ownership of artificial hip expertise lies in orthopaedics and device manufacturers.

The analysis in this chapter shows an integration of evidentiality into purchasing processes for the NHS. Analysis of the composition of the data evaluation panel in the national purchasing agency, for example, shows the pre-eminence of orthopaedic surgeons. The profession has become enrolled into a self-regulatory position. The purchasing agency has enrolled a significant commitment to data supply by manufacturers, though there are question marks against its potential regulatory effects.

In the UK, the Capital incident has led to stronger institutional and discursive links between the clinical science world and the world of medical device standards and centralised reporting and vigilance systems. The EU medical device regulations alone may not avoid the possibility of 'me-too' devices, requiring less thorough evaluation than substantially new devices entering the marketplace, although the reclassification to a higher level of risk with increased requirement for marketing approval review should provide some counterbalance.

The recent history of artificial hips and their regulation, as with breast implants, illustrates an increase in the plurality of constituencies and modes of influence shaping regulatory activity. There have been calls to increase long-term randomised controlled trials of total hip prostheses in spite of the high rate of technological innovation. A number of HTA agencies in Europe have investigated these issues (Pons et al., 1999). HTA has been engaged in nationally distinct projects to reduce scientific uncertainty about the financial and health risk of this technology. Here, therefore, we see regulatory science in action, orchestrated by the state in conjunction with clinical scientists active in healthcare delivery. HTA analysis highlighted the fact that most evidence about THR performance has been produced by specialist surgeons working in research-intensive healthcare provider organisations, notably teaching hospitals. Surgeons in such centres were more likely to have vested interest in demonstrating good results and to have more resources to invest in prosthesis-specific training programmes and the like. Arguably, this problem in producing robust orthopaedic knowledge has been recognised and countered by the institution of the NJR in the UK, which at the time of writing is close to comprehensive in collating data from its target hospitals.

Even where a medical device is regarded as highly successful, there are a number of issues of uncertainty. Healthcare risk and the implications of these devices for public health are matters of negotiation among competing groups. In the European context the regulatory environment is becoming more complex and, in principle, more stringent especially with regard to vigilance systems. However, the effectiveness of vigilance systems for the timely identification of under-performing devices is in question. Some areas of uncertainty, such as the definition of 'novelty' have been identified. Public policy–related healthcare science has focused upon the issues of clinical and cost-effectiveness on the basis of comparative clinical research on the longevity of implants and economic analysis. A viewpoint of implantees is conspicuously absent in these approaches.

The use of registries has emerged as a key development in the governance of artificial hips. The NJR combines technological data on different prosthesis designs with societal data about the organisational actors in the healthcare system. The way in which this extremely detailed data source will be developed and what sort of knowledge will be produced from it is not clear. At present there is no evidence of significant achievement of the governance aim of containing or reducing the proliferation of different models of artificial hip technology.

Artificial hip technology and society

Artificial hip technology has reached a plateau in its innovation pathway. There is limited sign of technological standardisation (Faulkner, 2002; Neary, 2007). It is tempting to draw the easy conclusion that the highly diversified marketplace of hip prostheses is the outcome of biological, technological and societal complexity. Indeed, the case study supports this broad and rather vague conclusion. But in this final discussion I consider the conundrum of technology and society in the case of the innovation pathway of artificial hips in greater detail. In particular I point to the applicability of notions of medicalisation, the construction of usership and the shaping of technology, medicine-industry-state-science dynamics and legitimation.

In artificial hip technology we have witnessed one of the most celebrated achievements of technological medicine being also the subject of one of the most extreme interrogations by the regulatory state. The production of evidence for hip technology has mushroomed. The technical science of technological performance plays a large part in the case study, healthcare science has also been very prominent, and latterly the co-ordination of national-level monitoring processes has become pre-eminent. It has been necessary to describe aspects of the material technology in some detail in order to convey its importance to the associated processes of innovation and governance.

The concept of medicalisation applied to medical technology requires a consideration of the 'social nature' of the material technology. The social experience and meanings of artificial hips are not easily accessible in public or patient domains. Hip prostheses *per se* are not information-rich technologies; the information that end-users and the public obtain are mediated through science, surveillance and clinical encounters produced by a variety of organised groups and agencies of health professionals, public health and health technology assessors and regulators. Similarly, access to information about the range of prosthetic designs and materials in the marketplace is limited to those with specialist knowledge and interest. Biophysical complexity and variation of the population is not simply reflected in the proliferation of different types and variants of hip technology. Nor is it clear that medico-industrial innovation and marketing is the sole driver. As this case study shows, between these two extremes there has been an evidence-fuelled struggle between innovating forces and regulating forces.

The societally medicalising significance of artificial hips as a form of medical intervention is low. This means that other theories that try to apply notions of consumption and active, participatory, technology-shaping participation to the society/technology conundrum also have little purchase. Domestication theory makes little sense here, unless we use it metaphorically to conceptualise bodies of the individuals biological acceptance and interaction with the prosthesis. This is not to say that the designers, producers, marketers and sellers of contemporary hip technologies do not do work that may configure end-users in particular ways. Indeed the advertising of hip prostheses is conspicuous in promoting images of a 'natural' paradigm of biocompatibility and 'ingrowth' of manufactured material into human bone, suggesting a literal normalisation of prosthetic technology in the human population. The brand names of prostheses such as 'BioGroove Hip System' and 'Natural-Fit' emphasise the appeal to nature, flexibility and choice. However, the user being addressed in such processes is the surgeon rather than the patient.

The usership of hip technologies is dominated by orthopaedic surgeons. This dominance is an accomplishment rather than a given fact. It has been achieved partly through professional organisation and activism, representation in governance developments that I have described, and partly by the close interdependence of the specialised practices of orthopaedic surgery and the material technologies which surgeons use. Orthopaedic surgeons have been involved in a major process of negotiation with the other key stakeholder groups that have mobilised and become active in this field. The analysis of science and governance has shown the growth of the production of evidence amidst concern and controversy about the methodological criteria for producing it. It has shown also the development of closer linkage between evidence-production and regulatory agencies – much of which has been orchestrated by the healthcare state – in a form of regulatory evidentiality.

It has been noted that safety and efficacy are often constituted in different 'nodes of the network that constitutes the social system of medical care' (Bodewitz et al., 1987). The HTA scientific agenda broadened the participation in efficacy/effectiveness evaluation to include constituencies outside the orthopaedic profession, notably independent healthcare evaluators such as clinical epidemiologists and health economists. The evidence-based movements here have 'brought the State in' to the evaluation of medical practice. The profession-led investigation of the Capital incident is an example of the enrolment of evidentiality into processes of accountability and legitimation that translate 'internal' issues of healthcare system risk – complexity, confusion, cost, safety, efficacy, expertise – beyond the boundaries of the healthcare system into 'external' issues susceptible to governance and debate in the public sphere. The new institutions of evidence-appraisal, especially the NICE in the UK, are positioned so that this public forum–defining effect can be achieved.

The analysis of governance here shows strong evidence of the existence of a medico-industrial complex in which clinical practitioners and manufacturers are closely, if uneasily, bound together and of a form of relationship between industry and state that can be described as conforming to a corporatist model. Governance attempts to control the gatekeeping of hip prostheses from a public health perspective must be regarded as mild (van der Meulen, 2005). The 'gold standard' ideology of the randomised control trial has been joined in the 2000s by institutions of regulatory evidentiality focused on surveillance and monitoring. Interestingly, the surveillance dataset–based model of evaluation is 'post-modernist' in the sense that it goes beyond the gold standard of the RCT, even though critics may continue to espouse that model as the pinnacle of methodological rigour (cf. van der Meulen, 2005). One of the reasons for this lies with the 'social nature' of the technology as an invisible, long-lifetime technology best assessed by long-term studies, but which nevertheless requires short-term performance results for safety assessment to be produced.

The orthopaedic profession has been fighting a rearguard self-regulatory action around artificial hips. A re-legitimation of total hip replacement has been sought, with a major focus upon an essentially modernist marshalling of evidence, in order to maintain the credibility of hip replacement both inside the healthcare system and in the wider society. In this process the state has assumed a rather adversarial mode of engagement with orthopaedics and has tried to strengthen its resistance to industrial powers of innovation and diffusion. Technological success has thus been followed by a diversification of innovation pathways evoking a remarkably high level of multiplication of regulatory surveillance in recent years, whose effectiveness, nevertheless, is yet to be demonstrated.

5

The PSA Test for Prostate Cancer: Risk Constructs Governance?

Introduction

> A new generation of tests for cancer could do more harm than good by increasingly diagnosing tumours which may not pose an immediate health risk, according to a leading cancer specialist.
>
> (*Guardian*, 3 April 2007)

> Use of the PSA test is swamping urology and radiotherapy services, the Government's cancer tsar has admitted.
>
> (UK newspaper report, 2006)

The PSA test is a technology developed in the 1980s, first used to assist in the monitoring of, and subsequently also in the detection of prostate cancer. It is not on its own a diagnostic test. Regulatory regimes classify it as an *in vitro* medical device. It is a blood test. Following consultation and ordering of the test from a medical professional, analysis conventionally is conducted in a pathology laboratory. 'Home test' kits can, however, be purchased in the burgeoning do-it-yourself healthcare marketplace. The prostate is a small gland found only in men which is important to sexual and reproductive functioning, having a role in liquefying sperm at the time of ejaculation. The result of testing indicates the possible presence of a protein unique to the prostate and associated at above-normal levels with potential pathology.

Prostate cancer is a potentially serious and in some cases life-threatening disease. Many cases are asymptomatic. It emerged as a high profile subject, newsworthy in the public media, during the 1990s.

Media headlines such as 'Rising fear of prostate cancer "could cost the NHS £400m"' (*Guardian*, 31 October 1995) were common. It was, and continues to be common to hear about public figures who had contracted the disease, such as the US General Norman Schwarzkopf, the musician Frank Zappa and the British comedian Bob Monkhouse. Such personalised references undoubtedly raised the public profile of the disease and increased the public perception of its risks. Media accounts are frequently controversial.

Prostate cancer and the detection of it are high stakes issues for men, and for healthcare evidence and policy. The detection of prostate cancer can be regarded as going to the heart of issues akin to the environmental risks conjured up in the notion of the 'risk society' (Beck, 1992). As will be seen in this chapter, prostate cancer involves not only high stakes but also risks characterised by high uncertainty – scientific, professional, political and personal.

The detection and treatment of localised prostate cancer has attracted more funding from the UK's national HTA research programme than any other single subject. It is thus of the highest possible priority in terms of the production of healthcare knowledge. Many other healthcare policy agencies internationally have conducted major investigations of the same topic. Experimental studies in the US and Europe have involved the recruitment of several hundred thousand men in various strategies to answer questions about screening, detection and treatment. Government policy on prostate cancer detection has been raised as an issue of public importance several times in debates in the British Parliament. Screening in particular continues to be a much-debated issue. PSA testing for prostate cancer can be seen, as alluded to in the newspaper report quoted at the beginning of this chapter, as being in the vanguard of the wider development of cancer tests using new whole-body scanning techniques and genetic tests which will identify small, latent and frequently benign cancerous cells and tissue.

The risks related to the PSA test and to prostate cancer are various. They concern not only the disease itself, but also men's anxieties about the knowledge provided by the test, actual side effects of treatments and risks associated with scientific investigation of the use of the test. Cancer-related trials may pose direct risks of safety and efficacy for participating patients (Keating & Cambrosio, 2006). The representation of clinical trials in the sociomedical sphere may amplify awareness of risks. As discussed in Chapter 2, the deployment of detection and screening technologies is part of a societal and healthcare system process that defines the contours of citizens' experience of risks.

The case of PSA testing is the subject of continuing public debate and controversy, therefore attracting a wider range of stakeholders and higher levels of concern than many technologies; the PSA test applies – directly – only to men, bringing gender issues into consideration; the disease involved is a life-threatening cancer, but unlike some cancers there is no clear-cut therapeutic pathway for localised (gland-confined) occurrences; by any standards of the healthcare sciences, the volume of the global production of evidence about PSA testing is massive, and the nature of some of the science designed in this field in the UK, as will be seen, is innovative; and the linkages between public policy and the delivery and consumption of PSA testing are complicated and tendentious.

The chapter is more concerned with the practices, organisational and interpretative, of PSA testing rather than the material technology *per se*. Crucial to the techno-practice of PSA testing is the notion of a *cut-off point* on the gauge showing the PSA level in the blood, above which normal functioning may be deemed suspect. This can be likened to the speed limit for motor cars and the social practices of car driving. There is a limit above which the working of the car itself is at risk, but there are lower limits which may be normatively defined for social and public health and safety reasons, sanctioned by regulations, and these may well be disputed and contravened by practitioners.

This chapter, therefore, discusses the sociomedical innovation space of PSA testing. It focuses on the dynamics of the emergence and uptake of the testing technology in practice, its routinisation as a more or less stable, collective, but variably patterned medical practice, its users, promoters and opponents, the production of evidence about prostate cancer detection by the healthcare sciences and how it has figured in evidence-related policymaking. As indicated in this introduction, PSA technology and its interpretation carry their own peculiar forms of risk. The chapter examines the question of how the construction of PSA-related risks is related to societal governance, and the positioning of the healthcare sciences in governance processes. Apart from published data, it draws on my experience in national HTA during the 1990s, interviews with key participants and archival research in the Centre for the History of Evaluation in Health Care (CHEHC) at Cardiff University.

Epidemiology and the marketplace

Prostate cancer is a significant health problem with significant mortality rates. The epidemiology of the disease itself is not fully detailed here but some key data are presented in order to give an indication of its prevalence and incidence. It is worth noting at the outset one recurrent comment among clinical and epidemiological scientists engaged with this disease – that most men die *with* it rather than *from* it. Thus we note some advisory precaution in interpreting the true 'size of the problem' for society. For example, statements from stakeholders wishing to emphasise the importance of the problem, such as it being 'the most commonly *diagnosed* cancer in men', need to be interpreted in this light. Diagnosis does not translate straightforwardly into symptoms or progression.

The incidence of detection rose dramatically during the 1980s and early 1990s internationally, while rates of mortality have risen slightly over the last 20 years. Perhaps contrary to popular belief, incidence rates peaked in the late 1990s. In 2005 the deaths of 10,000 men were attributed to prostate cancer in the UK, a crude rate of 34 per 100,000, and an age-standardised rate (against European benchmarks) of 25.4 per 100,000. It is the second most common cause of cancer *mortality* among men, after lung cancer, and in men over age 85 it is the most common. Autopsy investigations show that at this age and over, the great majority of men have some signs of the disease localised in the prostate. Death rates overall rise with increasing age.

It has been clear that part of the upward trend in incidence should be attributed to increased rates of detection. There is some uncertainty about trends around the late 1980s to early 1990s in the industrialised countries. In spite of a general upward trend in most countries, there were inconsistencies in the relationship between increasing PSA rates and increasing mortality rates across a wide range of countries. There were claims especially in the US that the increasing and extensive use of PSA testing was leading to a reduction in mortality rates associated with early treatments, but these and other epidemiological data suggested that this conclusion was premature (Oliver et al., 2001). It remains impossible to identify how much of the recent fall in mortality is the result of factors such as PSA testing, improvements in treatment, changes in cancer registration practices or the way in which deaths are attributed to prostate cancer. Importantly, prostate cancer rates vary between different ethnic groups. Its incidence is relatively low in some Asian populations, especially Japanese, and relatively high among men of African-Caribbean extraction, a phenomenon that occurs on both sides of the Atlantic and is the subject of continuing epidemiological and genetic investigation. Apart from race, other possible risk factors are thought to include a diet high in animal fats and proteins, and a family history of the disease is known to increase the risk.

Public and media representations of prostate cancer and the PSA test's role in it tend towards hyperbole and confusion. For example, in September 2007, Roger Kirby, a well known campaigning urological surgeon, chair of the Prostate Research Campaign charity, and in favour of active therapy, was quoted thus: 'Expert says males should show a feminine, less career-driven side to cut prostate disease risk' (Hill, 2007). The article evoked an outraged response, including one from the former editor of the *British Medical Journal*, who said 'Red-blooded, money-making, over-worked, stressed alpha males get prostate cancer, while "new men" fade away with something effete. Unfortunately it's all non-sense' (Smith, 2007). Such exchanges in the public sphere indicate the highly divergent and emotive views that abound.

It remains, of course, that prostate cancer is a serious disease with high mortality rates, but in order to understand its controversial pathway through healthcare, we must look at how the PSA test is used in medical practice, what information about it is disseminated to citizens and to clinicians and how policy communities attempt to control it and shape the healthcare science of which its detection is part.

Development of the PSA test

Before the development of the PSA test, doctors had even less means to detect prostate cancer. Digital rectal examination (DRE) was used with limited success, otherwise symptomatic and opportunistic diagnosis took place. During the 1970s, researchers demonstrated that prostate-specific proteins, such as PSA, are released from prostate cells during the course of tumor development (Wang et al., 1979). These early developments suggested that PSA could be used as a treatment marker, and possibly a diagnostic tool. Several biomedical manufacturers have made the PSA blood test widely available. In 1986, it was approved by the US Food and Drug Administration for use as a monitoring test for treatment and disease recurrence, the first regulatory authority worldwide to do so, and in 1994 it was further approved as an aid for early detection of the disease.

Industry involvement in developing the basic PSA technology and emerging variants has been strong. The most widely used technology continues to be produced by Hybritech Inc., a San Diego, USA-based firm that was bought by the global pharmaceutical company Eli Lilly in 1985. Hybritech was the first and one of the most financially successful of the specialised biotechnology companies in the US. The commercially available PSA assays use several different biochemical techniques, raising issues of standardisation. Variants to the basic PSA test continue to be developed. There are a large number of studies assessing the relative merits of the various newer developments of the technology. Most PSA is bound to proteins, but some is free-floating. In the early 1990s it was discovered that measuring the ratio of 'free' to 'total' PSA could help distinguish prostate cancer from benign prostate disease (Free/total PSA). The emergence of 'free' PSA testing means that the original PSA test is now often referred to as 'total PSA'.

Following recent scientific doubt about the PSA test, even among some of its American originators (Stamey et al., 2004), high-profile urologists have leapt to its defence: 'PSA and Free-PSA Testing for Prostate Cancer Is Still a Lifesaver' (Catalona, et al., 2005). The authors state that while understanding of the total PSA test continues to evolve, 'the PSA test is even more specific than mammograms are for detecting early-stage breast cancer'.

PSA test interpretation

The calibration of PSA is key to its use. The presence of the antigen in serum blood is conventionally expressed in terms of nanograms per millilitre (ng/mL), a 'normal' level being either 3 or 4 ng/ml. The interpretation of this figure is important and disputed. Technologically, the problem with the widely used total PSA test is that it does not have a good predictive value – thus a 'positive' test does not necessarily indicate a cancer which will go on to become symptomatic, nor does a 'negative' result necessarily rule out cancer. Known reasons for individual raised PSA are: pathological prostate cancer, benign prostatic hypertrophy (BPH), urine infection; ejaculation in the previous 48 hours, recent vigorous exercise such as riding a bike, a prostate biopsy in the past six months and digital rectal examination in the previous week. In the UK, the NICE also expressed concerns about the application of the test:

> a quarter to a third of men with PSA over 10 ng/ml have prostate cancer but PSA levels vary widely, both among men who do have cancer and those who do not. There is no criterion below which men may be reassured that they do not have cancer, nor an agreed level which is regarded as diagnostic. Different systems for measuring PSA can produce quite variable results and apparent changes in PSA levels can reflect the use of assay materials from different manufacturers.
>
> (NICE, 2002)

This situation is compounded by the fact that in spite of there being three major modes of treatment for the localised prostate-confined disease, the one to prefer in general or in individual cases is unknown. Clinical practitioners and industry acknowledge the indicative rather than definitive nature of the PSA test. While it appears that undergoing the test is itself 'risky' and the information (or, rather, data) it provides difficult to understand, it is important to examine evidence indicating users' experiences, beliefs and expectations. This issue is tackled in the following section.

Usership, expertise and experience

Usership of the PSA test is more difficult to define even than for the other technologies discussed in this book. This is because the emphasis is on the interpretative practices associated with it rather then the device itself. The healthcare practices associated with the test, and the activity of urologists and GPs in particular, are discussed in the following section. Here I focus on the experience of men as consumers of it.

Men's experience

Evidence of men's experience of the PSA test can be gathered from a variety of sources. I am relying here largely upon secondary sources, and I refer to methodological issues in citing specific sources. In particular, this section includes reference to research undertaken in the Health Services Research (HSR) scientific paradigm, that produces evidence about 'quality of life'. The high public profile of the test and the disease means that representations of men's experience percolate into the public domain frequently, and this also is a source of evidence. Because of the many controversies involved, occasions for mass media attention are also frequently occasions for stakeholders such as cancer charities and scientific investigators to pronounce publicly upon their views.

It appears from a recently published review that the knowledge of prostate cancer detection is low in the general population. Men do not possess 'basic knowledge' about prostate screening and prostate cancer in the US and a range of European countries according to an international study (cited in Hewitson and Austoker, 2005). The study found that 22 per cent of men in the UK were aware of the PSA test and only one per cent were aware that prostate cancer could be asymptomatic. The review authors regard the knowledge of PSA testing and prostate cancer as 'relatively poor', and this 'highlights the need [for the UK's Prostate Cancer Risk Management Programme (PCRMP) – referred to in more detail in Policy and Governance section below] to disseminate information about PSA testing and the importance for this information to be of the highest possible standard' (Hewitson and Austoker, 2005).

The PSA test in the context of prostate cancer is one of the areas that Database of Individual Patient Experience (DIPEx) has chosen for attention.[1] This resource has assembled a set of accounts by men who have encountered the technology, based on 42 interviews. DIPEx's own summary of the experiences includes:

> Men's experiences of making decisions about the PSA test reflect the uncertainty about the benefits of the test. Some saw it as a routine test, as 'responsible health behaviour' ... and recommended that other men their age should consider it, but others emphasised that it is less straightforward than a cholesterol or blood pressure check and that men need to be fully informed and prepared for the consequences if their results are 'abnormal'.
>
> (DIPEx.org, 2007)

The oral and video evidence of DIPEx indicates that there is huge variation in the views of men. Reaching age 50 had prompted some men to ask for a test, but in other cases men had declined following discussion with a GP. One man's experience was summarised: 'He had the PSA test primarily to humour his urologist. The result left him feeling extremely anxious, and he wished he had talked to a trained counsellor' beforehand. The possible significance of the PSA test may not always be apparent to men undergoing it: 'For him the PSA test was no problem whatsoever; he went to work five minutes later' (DIPEx.org).

Further evidence has been provided by a qualitative interview-based study, which investigated 28 men who had undertaken a PSA test in a primary care setting (Evans et al., 2007). Ages were between 40 and 75 years, 20/28 had urological symptoms and thus might have been expected to be better informed than the general population. One of the strengths of this study is that it investigates PSA in the 'natural' context of day-to-day health service primary care. Unsurprisingly with a relatively small sample and as the authors acknowledge, key groups were unrepresented in the sample, namely men who had declined to undergo the test when it was offered and men from minority ethnic groups. Concluding that men's PSA decision is influenced generally by an amalgam of 'social' and 'media' contextual factors, one of the main findings of this research was that the experience of uncertainty could persist even after a 'normal' test result. The men in this South Wales sample commented on their 'lay referral networks'. One asymptomatic man with a brother who had had 'prostate trouble' said:

> (My brother) said that it could be hidden and you don't know it's there. So he badgered me for quite a long time.
>
> (from Evans et al., 2007)

This man had a raised PSA and prostate cancer was diagnosed. Similarly, men were aware of mass media representations of the disease, especially through newspapers. In the same research, uncertainties of the PSA test were another major theme. Men differed in their understandings of this. One man with symptoms said that: 'it's a "maybe" test. Maybe you have maybe you haven't'. Some men found it difficult to understand the message that PSA test results were not necessarily specific to prostate cancer – because it can also indicate benign prostate enlargement. There was some understanding of the metaphor that some cancers are 'tigers' and others are 'pussycats' not needing active treatment. As with other asymptomatic conditions, some men expressed the view that they 'don't want to know'. The possible massive impact of a raised PSA test on men was evoked: 'I had seen things on the internet that a PSA of around 20 was not good. To think I got double this. I was very worried' (from Evans et al., 2007).

It appears overall that men subsequently diagnosed with localised prostate cancer, perhaps unsurprisingly, are in favour of PSA testing and a policy of screening for the disease (Chapple et al., 2002). The issue of 'need to know' versus 'not wanting to know' was highlighted as a dilemma in a medical programme broadcast by the BBC in the UK in the mid-2000s. (BBC Radio 4, 2006; a series called 'Am I Normal?' that investigated normality and identity in physical or medical conditions of contemporary public concern). A prostate cancer specialist noted:

> if you've got a 'nice' prostate cancer that doesn't need treatment, it's better not to know ... unfortunately nowadays we're finding a lot of those nice prostate cancers, and then having to live with the knowledge that we've got them – for 20 or 30 years.

The programme included an account from a man who had had a PSA test with a positive result at the age of 57. His account, remarkably, shows that the advice he received about the appropriate action to take, from different physicians, started with surgery, moved to radiotherapy, and then to an offer of participation in an 'active surveillance' programme. The regime required the PSA blood test every three months and a biopsy every two years. It turned out in his account that 'Clive' had had a PSA value of 4.5 ng/mL, which many clinicians would regard as scarcely above normal. This raised the question of how clinical specialists, trained to treat cancer therapeutically, might influence men's knowledge and decisions. The specialist involved with active surveillance noted that 'in my experience patients are more open to active surveillance than some clinicians'. 'Clive' said that he thinks everyone is increasingly 'living with' cancer and that 'we will call it something else'. He concluded that: 'I *have* cancer but I don't *suffer* from it', starkly emphasising the ambiguity and ambivalence in his experience of citizenship and patienthood: 'I am not a "cancer patient" – but I am a cancer patient' (BBC Radio 4, 2006).

The DIPEx resource mentioned above also supplies examples of what we can call, following a classic sociological/anthropological paper (Davison et al., 1991), the lay epidemiology of the PSA test–prostate cancer mortality association. Thus one man shared his interpretation of epidemiological statistics:

> There have been examples of screening which has proved highly successful in the Austrian Tyrol for example, the screening for over 60,000 men was offered free on a 5 year period. As a result of this, deaths from prostate cancer fell by 43% whereas in other cantons of Austria where this screening was not offered death rate remained exactly the same.
>
> (DIPEx.org; Prostate Cancer – Interview 34)

The Austrian Tyrol research is quite widely quoted in public health debates. The interpretation should not, however, be taken at face value. Due to the phenomenon of 'lead time bias', the association between PSA testing and mortality rates is by no means clear from the figures cited: the earlier diagnoses facilitated by the PSA test mean that cancers are detected earlier and the rate of detection is higher. In this circumstance, unless the underlying disease suddenly becomes more aggressive in the population generally, the rate of mortality is bound to reduce, given a steady state in the effectiveness of treatments.

'Quality of life'

Some HSR projects have attempted to investigate men's experience of PSA testing using conventional quality-of-life measurement tools such as the HADS (Hospital Anxiety and Depression Score) and the SF-36, probably the most widely used 'activities of daily living' instrument in worldwide healthcare research. One such study, for example, in this case linked to the

ProtecT trial discussed later in this chapter, concluded that: 'the deleterious effects of receiving an abnormal PSA result during population screening are not identified by generic health-status questionnaires' (Brindle et al., 2006). This is an interesting and counter-intuitive conclusion when considered in the face of the rich qualitative accounts provided in interviews and personal testimonies, illustrated above. Given that HSR/HTA is closely tied to processes of healthcare governance and regulation, I return to the products of such research in the section below ('Science').

Advocacy

In the UK, the Consumers Association is the major national non-statutory organisation providing advice and information on consumer products, famous for its '*Which?*' reports. There was a '*Health Which?*' equivalent and this examined self-test kits, including those for prostate cancer, in 2002. Under the humorous title 'Don't try these at home', the basic message was clear:

> Our experts agreed that people would be seriously affected by the knowledge of a positive result, even though the manufacturers make no direct association between the tests and prostate cancer. Our oncologist advised that people should always see their GP first.
>
> (Consumers Association 2002)

Interestingly the UK's independent Men's Health Forum has not been an advocate of screening or individual detection using the PSA test. They have taken a cautious position, essentially advising men to consult their GP. They do suggest that men who are at greater risk, with a family history of prostate cancer, and men of Afro-Caribbean descent should think about it more actively (cited in Roberts, 2004).

This chapter has already suggested that advocacy of the PSA test by the medical professions themselves is a very controversial and contested issue. This is considered further in the following section, which discusses evidence of the use of the PSA test within the healthcare system, and the attitudes of medical practitioners towards it.

Healthcare practice – diffusion of the PSA test

Diffusion of the PSA test in the UK is widespread, but the evidence of this is not robust. It is known that PSA test rates have increased in primary care in England and Wales. In 2004 a six per cent overall rate of testing was reported; this included a two per cent rate in asymptomatic men, which would have been higher if private testing (outside the NHS) were included (Melia et al., 2004). Rates of testing decrease with higher levels of socioeconomic deprivation. The exact proportion of asymptomatic men being tested, and the extent to which this is patient-driven, is unknown. In men in England and Wales aged over 45 years in 1994 with no previous diagnosis, 1.4 per cent were tested per annum; in 1999, 3.5 per cent were tested per annum; in 2001–2 this had increased to 5.4 per cent (Melia, 2005).

Further indication of diffusion is provided from an online self-report survey of 400 GPs (Brett et al., 2005). GPs were given vignettes of men with LUTS (lower urinary tract syndrome) and a family history of cancer, and of men asymptomatic but requesting PSA having 'lost a friend' to prostate cancer. The study provided some confirmation that PSA testing in asymptomatic men is a regular occurrence in the UK, and that there is general support from GPs for the policy of making PSA tests available to 'informed' men. It has been suggested by randomised control study that educational interventions with physicians can 'improve' (that is, reduce) deployment of the test (Weller et al., 2003).

Turning from general practice to the medical specialties, in the late 1990s the practices of urological surgeons using the PSA test were surveyed in conjunction with a national Health Technology Assessment systematic review (Faulkner et al., 2000). The extent of variation in clinical practice with the PSA test would have direct implications for the pattern and volume of further diagnostic activity and treatment. The survey considered beliefs and practice primarily among urologists. The study concluded that urological centres where there was a urologist specialising in prostate cancer were more likely to use lower cut-off points in interpreting PSA levels, thus making it more likely that further action would follow in these centres (Faulkner et al., 2000). Thus it was highly likely that aspects of the organisation of urological services, which vary between geographical areas and healthcare centres, and the socialisation of urologists led to an unequal social patterning of detection of the disease among men in the UK.

This variation was paralleled in research that revealed variations in type and approach to treatment of localised prostate cancer. A survey of oncologists had shown that they would generally treat with radiotherapy rather than surgery, a more conservative approach (Savage et al., 1997). However, in spite of relative conservatism in the UK, there were rapid increases in the use of surgery – radical prostatectomy – in England during the 1990s in urologists' reported preferences for treatment options

(Donovan et al., 1999), confirmed by NHS data that showed an upward trend, though with marked regional variations possibly related to access to PSA testing and the location of surgeons (Oliver et al., 2003).

In the UK, private health companies like BUPA routinely offer PSA testing to men over the age of 50 as part of 'wellman' checks. In a newspaper report the clinical director of BUPA Wellness presented this picture, which, as shown above, may not do justice to the actual variation in men's views and practices:

> Before offering men routine screening for prostate cancer, we ensure that they are informed of the pros and cons of testing. Ninety per cent of them have the test. ... Where we find an illness, people are very grateful that it has been caught early. Where nothing is found, people are relieved.
>
> (Roberts, 2004)

So there is evidence that PSA test rates have been increasing in the UK, and in some centres, rates of surgery as well. As the newspaper quotation at the beginning of the chapter indicated, there is political concern that these upward trends are putting a burden on health services that cannot be met. The impact on healthcare resources is difficult to ascertain clearly, but 'Urologists report seeing many more patients with possible prostate cancer, and expect to see even more in the future' (NICE, 2002).

Ideally, I would include here information about the self-testing rates of men who undertake the PSA test using commercial self-test kits. However, there are few data in the UK to assess this, and this is clearly a gap in the research record. One study based on a small sample of general practices, ongoing at the time of writing, has been described (Wilson et al., 2006). It is clear here that the level of clinical concern about cancer-related self-testing is high. Test kits can be obtained readily, for example from community pharmacists and online shops. Some test kits provide the total PSA value in an onscreen display. There is no doubt that overall rates of self-testing for a variety of conditions are rising. Sales of self-testing equipment generally are reported to have increased dramatically: over £54m was spent on self-diagnostic products in the UK in 2002 according to market research, a 32 per cent increase since 1998 (newspaper report cited by Wilson et al., op. cit.). A survey of self-test kits available through the Internet to UK consumers found in 2006 that there were 4 kits available giving immediate readouts of PSA, and one providing the result via a laboratory (Ryan et al., 2006).

In summary, the evidence about the practice of PSA testing in the UK healthcare system is that although medical practitioners subscribe to a view of 'informing the patient' in this field, the extent and nature of information-sharing is unknown, and observable rates of PSA testing and of radical treatment once cancer is diagnosed, are rising.

Science

Healthcare science

Prostate cancer screening was identified as one of the highest priorities in the first research agenda of the UK national HTA programme. In the mid-1990s this HTA programme commissioned two largely quantitative 'systematic reviews' (Chamberlain et al., 1997; Selley et al., 1997). The reviews considered hundreds of studies of the performance of PSA tests and its variants and concluded that there was inadequate evidence to support the introduction of mass screening. These conclusions, as the UK government stated, were subsequently supported by HTA reports from several other countries (eight reports from seven countries were produced, according to the International Association of Health Technology Assessment organisations). Awareness of the conclusions 'helped to contain the uncontrolled dissemination of PSA testing' – a statement whose fragility is demonstrated in this chapter. In fact, the two systematic reviews were taken as an opportunity by the chair of the then new national Standing Group on Health Technology to highlight the new HTA movement with a clear, evidence-based message. A public and media launch for the reports proved controversial especially among cancer charities and some urological surgeons who objected to the cautious message on screening.

It was clear that there was a need to communicate evidence to medical communities and to patients/citizens in different formats. The newly founded NHS Centre for Reviews and Dissemination produced publications about PSA testing and prostate cancer for all GPs in England and Wales, and for any man who requested it. The former was presented in the series of *'Effective Health Care Bulletins'* and the latter in the series *'Effectiveness Matters'*, illustrated in Figure 5.1. It is clear that the uncertainty confirmed by the HTA science was to be shared with GPs and with men. The primary advice was that health professionals should discuss with patients the evidence of the risks of prostate cancer, its treatment and its detection via PSA. In other words, there was a move towards a 'counselling' mode of shared decision-making enshrined in healthcare policy, based on HTA. Tellingly, cancer charities' requests for their contact details to be included in these documents were declined.

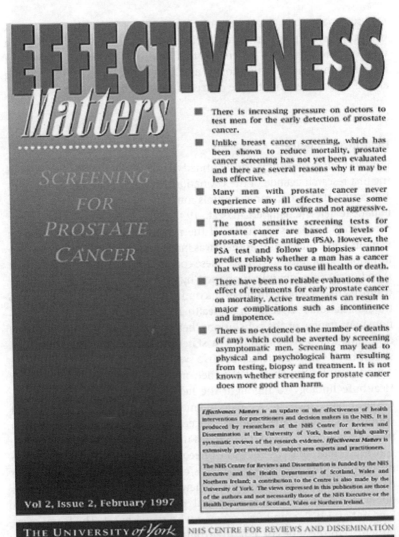

EFFECTIVENESS
Matters

SCREENING
FOR
PROSTATE
CANCER

- There is increasing pressure on doctors to test men for the early detection of prostate cancer.

- Unlike breast cancer screening, which has been shown to reduce mortality, prostate cancer screening has not yet been evaluated and there are several reasons why it may be less effective.

- Many men with prostate cancer never experience any ill effects because some tumours are slow growing and not aggressive.

- The most sensitive screening tests for prostate cancer are based on levels of prostate specific antigen (PSA). However, the PSA test and follow up biopsies cannot predict reliably whether a man has a cancer that will progress to cause ill health or death.

- There have been no reliable evaluations of the effect of treatments for early prostate cancer on mortality. Active treatments can result in major complications such as incontinence and impotence.

- There is no evidence on the number of deaths (if any) which could be averted by screening asymptomatic men. Screening may lead to physical and psychological harm resulting from testing, biopsy and treatment. It is not known whether screening for prostate cancer does more good than harm.

Effectiveness Matters is an update on the effectiveness of health interventions for practitioners and decision makers in the NHS. It is produced by researchers at the NHS Centre for Reviews and Dissemination at the University of York, based on high quality systematic reviews of the research evidence. *Effectiveness Matters* is extensively peer reviewed by subject area experts and practitioners.

The NHS Centre for Reviews and Dissemination is funded by the NHS Executive and the Health Departments of Scotland, Wales and Northern Ireland; a contribution to the Centre is also made by the University of York. The views expressed in this publication are those of the authors and not necessarily those of the NHS Executive or the Health Departments of Scotland, Wales or Northern Ireland.

Vol 2, Issue 2, February 1997

THE UNIVERSITY *of York*   NHS CENTRE FOR REVIEWS AND DISSEMINATION

Figure 5.1 Information leaflet giving evidence-based recommendations against screening for prostate cancer

Subsequent to this early UK HTA work, the national HTA Programme in the UK has devoted further large amounts of resources (some £13 million, later raised to £20 million) to a research programme with the aim of producing evidence on which to secure NHS policy, including both the screening question and the 'therapeutic limbo' (Brown and Webster, 2004: 51) of the uncertainty of treatments. This scientific study has attracted more HTA funding than any other single topic since the programme began. It is still under way at the time of writing. A Medical Research Council (MRC) trial of alternative treatments had already failed to recruit sufficient patients, for disputed reasons, but including the possible predilection of urological surgeons towards surgical intervention and clinical belief that men did not consent to randomisation in a trial, nor to 'wait-and-see' approaches to treatment. In the event an innovative feasibility study was conducted, part of which was a methodological trial to assess different techniques of recruitment of patients. 'Such approaches need to retain the essential principle of randomisation while incorporating more fully patients' perspectives and preferences' (Donovan et al., 1999). The study used qualitative methods to assess men's reasons for participation or non-participation in the study. British Association of Urological Surgeons' (BAUS) representatives were at the time not happy with the direction that this national-level research was taking: 'support at present is only to be given to an uncontrolled pilot study which cannot provide a definitive answer to the dilemmas surrounding screening, and indeed may delay a conclusion to this controversy' (Dearnaley 1999). However, the feasibility study eventually proved successful and the result was the massive 'ProtecT' trial (Donovan et al., 2002, 2003). This offered men the PSA test and sought sufficient numbers of men diagnosed with localised prostate cancer to evaluate alternative treatments. This has offered the PSA test to over 100,000 men aged 50 to 69 in the UK. There was an ethical concern that men offered the test should be fully informed about the test and possible treatment side effects, the favoured approach being that this should be in the context of professional face-to-face consultation, rather than the conventional information sheet and consent form. The final trial design required that staff discussing the PSA test with men should hold professional counselling qualifications.

This progression to a counselling model of informed decision-making for PSA has also been accompanied by, and indeed partly constructed by, a strand of healthcare science focusing on men's experience of the PSA test and knowledge about it. Substantive accounts of men's experience from self-reports and testimonies have been discussed above. Here I consider clinical research and HSR that has examined the decision-making involved, and the implications for men. There are two main lines of research, firstly on the effects of 'information' on men's attitudes to undergoing the test, and secondly a focus on the psychosocial impacts of the test. The studies in this sub-field have been reviewed in detail (Hewitson & Austoker, 2005). Concluding their review of information provision (e.g. leaflets, video, counselling), the authors find a *lack* of firm evidence partly due to many studies attempting to assess intention to be tested rather than actual test-related behaviour, as well as a general lack of UK-based studies. While information provision has been deemed generally to reduce the proportions of men interested in undergoing the test, this was markedly less strong when free testing was offered as part of research projects, thus 'considerable caution should be exercised when attempting to draw conclusive links between the role of information in improving knowledge in men considering the PSA test and the relationship between information provision and men's intention to have the PSA test' (Hewitson & Austoker, op. cit., p. 25).

Regarding the psychosocial effects of PSA testing, again the quality of evidence has appeared problematic. The research by Brindle et al., cited above, which showed that conventional Quality of Life measurement may not capture significant aspects of men's experience of PSA testing, suggests that study reports in this field should be treated with caution. For example, conclusions such as 'Prostate cancer screening may be viewed by men as a routine examination, and therefore does not cause significantly large increases in HRQoL (Health-Related Quality of Life) or anxiety levels' (Essink Bot et al., 1998), may not be reliable. As Hewitson and Austoker (2005) concluded in their review, there are several other methodological concerns, including a lack of well conducted, randomised, prospective evaluations and the fact that most studies' participants had previous experience of prostate cancer screening. These reviewers illustrate the close discursive linkage that has emerged between scientific uncertainty on the one hand and the counselling model of healthcare practice on the other:

> Given that the most uncertainty and lack of conclusive scientific evidence is related to the consequences of having the PSA test (e.g. the benefits of early detection, the effectiveness of prostate biopsy, doubt surrounding the impact that treatment may have on a man's quality of life, etc.) it is vital that men are fully informed of the possible ramifications that having a PSA test may hold.
>
> (Hewitson & Austoker, 2005)

This diffusion of uncertainty is reinforced in guidance produced by the UK's PCRMP programme. Among the guidance produced by its expert group was consideration of how to deal with men suffering from LUTS.

The following are among the conclusions: 'Experts disagree as to whether men with LUTS should "opt-in" or "opt-out" of the PSA test, but all agree about the importance of fully counselling these men about the test implications.' And men at risk should not be targeted for the test: 'until more evidence is available about screening for prostate cancer, active case finding of men with risk factors is not recommended' (Watson et al., 2002).

In conclusion, the healthcare science of prostate cancer detection has been conducted at a symbolically important level in the UK, as elsewhere. The scientific activity of HTA expanded during the 1990s with prostate cancer screening research as one of its most important strands. The move towards a counselling and shared-decision-making model of interaction between men and the healthcare systems, and between men and scientific research is evident. This turn to pastoral care, where healthcare and science have become engaged with men's subjective experience outside as well as inside medical frameworks, is evidence of an increasing integration of science and state healthcare policy in this field. It is to the development and significance of the various strands of regulatory policy in PSA testing technology that I now turn.

Policy and Governance

European medical device regulation – in vitro diagnostic devices

European Directives are based around the appraisal of risk. The In-Vitro Medical Device Directive (IVMDD) is one of the three EU device directives that cover medical device technologies' safety and efficacy assessment and placing on the market. The aims of the IVMDD are to provide patients, users and third parties with a high level of health protection, removal of trade barriers in Europe and harmonisation of *in vitro* diagnostic medical devices standards. The PSA test falls within its jurisdiction.

Most devices can be given a CE mark by 'self-declaration' by manufacturers, but there are exceptions. The IVMDD groups In Vitro Devices (IVDs) into four categories so that the level of regulatory control applied to an IVD will be proportionate to the degree of assessed risk. The PSA test is noted in a special list. HIV testing is classified in 'List A', and 'List B', to give an idea of the context, includes PSA and tests for chlamydia, blood sugar measurement (diabetes), rubella and trisomy 21 (Down's Syndrome). Products requiring Notified Body assessment include those in List B and all self-test devices. For List B devices the Notified Body should either carry out an audit of the manufacturer's quality assurance system, or undertake examination and verification of each batch or product, or carry out 'type testing' (MHRA, undated). Under the Directive, Notified Bodies should examine manufacturers' technical documentation and also post production 'experience' and 'user experience'.

Issues of product labelling and 'information', some of which are matters of formal regulation, are important in considering this technology because they provide the link between the operation of the material technology and usership practices. This is especially obvious in the case of self-testing PSA kits, which are not permitted to make claims about the diagnosis of prostate cancer, although their potential *contribution* to diagnosis may play a part in advertising. The labelling and information requirements of *in vitro* diagnostic device technologies have recently been the subject of further EU guidance, which focuses primarily on the medium by which information is made available by manufacturers or distributors to end-users (European Commission DG Enterprise & Industry, 2007).

It is difficult, in the absence of primary research, to assess in detail the implications of the IVMDD for the healthcare use and patient experience of PSA testing. It is known that different manufacturers' technologies are not as standardised to each other as they could be, and this represents a possible problem for end-users who might move between healthcare settings accessing different laboratory test facilities. The EU has some initiatives in this area, underpinned by the commitment to harmonisation of technical standards. Most obviously though, the high risk classification of the PSA test highlights the seriousness of the perceived risk of the technology. Given the high rates of false positive results, the societally defined 'safety' of the device is a very ambiguous quality, constructed not only, not even primarily, by the safety and technical standards regime of market approval processes but also through the workings of science, governance and men's participation that I examine in this chapter.

Cancer screening and prostate cancer detection

Screening for disease is a policy arena in its own right in the UK. Growing ethical, social and economic concerns about the risk of screening were signalled in the UK by the formation in 1996 of a national advisory group, the National Screening Committee (NSC), to advise government on all existing and new screening technologies and programmes. This immediately identified screening for prostate cancer as a priority topic for review. Healthcare science was enrolled into the process of policy development with the aim of providing a solid basis for policy decisions (Sherriff et al., 1998).

Testing and screening for disease are popular in contemporary society. In the case of life-threatening illnesses, the popular image is that diseases apprehended early have a better chance of being cured or ameliorated. However, it is also the case for some that the offer of testing in the absence of symptoms does not evoke a positive response. The major question for policymakers has been: should a mass screening programme, akin to that available for women in the case of breast and cervical cancer, be introduced? And the answer to this question in the UK, officially, and with the claimed support of extraordinarily detailed 'evidence', has been – and remains – a very firm 'not yet'. The absence of national screening programmes for men, compared to breast cancer and cervical screening for women in the UK, has been noted in public debate. The perception of this gender disadvantage (whether it *is* a disadvantage to health in this instance is of course open to doubt) was reflected also by some academic work (Cameron & Bernardes, 1998).

The professional specialty most concerned with the PSA prostate cancer detection issue is urology. In the late 1990s, around the same time as the emergence of the HTA research, the BAUS produced recommendations to constrain use of the PSA test. BAUS made a number of statements about the controversy in the late 1990s when the appropriate avenue for future research was being hotly debated. Its Working Group proposed that 'the unthinking use of PSA, especially in elderly men where it causes distress and anxiety, must be prevented. The role of urologists must be to cooperate with colleagues in other specialties to prevent totally inappropriate investigation ... and to ensure that in other circumstances PSA testing is only carried out after appropriate counselling' (Dearnaley et al., 1999). It is thus clear that, apart from the doubt about benefits in population life expectancy from introducing a screening programme, the other danger perceived by policymakers and professional activists has been a threat of uncontrolled diffusion of testing.

The public profile of cancer and prostate cancer in particular is such that it has several times been discussed in the proceedings of the British Parliament over recent years. In June 2004 the Committee of Public Accounts, a 'public spending watchdog', considered the issue. The National Director of Cancer emphasised the NHS Prostate Cancer Programme launched in 2000, which 'looked at research, it looked at better treatment and at early detection'. The first national-level advisory group on a specific cancer in the UK was for prostate cancer. In March 2005 the Committee considered 'Cancer: The Patient's Experience', taking oral evidence again from the Chief Executive of the

Department of Health and the National Director for Cancer. The Committee raised issues including self-help groups and other support to men. Women, interestingly, were said to constitute the majority of people calling self-help groups for advice about prostate cancer. The Committee expressed their perception that implementation of the counselling model was problematic ('Why are we letting them down in terms of counselling?').

The government has been challenged about population screening, and has provided an account of its wide-ranging activities in this field in a written parliamentary reply (17 March 2006) by health minister Winterton:

> The Government are committed to introducing a national population screening programme for prostate cancer if and when screening and treatment techniques are sufficiently well developed ... The Department is supporting the development of screening technology for prostate cancer by having a comprehensive research strategy.

The reply continued with a detailed reference to the ProtecT mega-trial mentioned above:

> It is important to note that in order for a screening technology to contribute to saving lives it is essential for there to be effective treatments for the disease detected. That is why the Department is funding a £20 million trial of treatments for prostate specific antigen (PSA) screen-detected early prostate cancer.

At least one MP (Fraser) stated that the government position was unacceptably passive, and also felt that information about the PSA test was inadequate, stating that

> It is particularly important with prostate cancer – where a choice of treatment or, indeed, the choice of whether to treat exists – that patients remain in control of their care. That requires adequate information both in primary care, where initial discussions take place, and later in hospital, at the time of diagnosis.

The reference to 'remaining in control of their care' points towards the self-care agenda, which is discussed in the following section of this chapter. In December 2006, Winterton again answered questions noting that the 'main driver' to improve prostate cancer services was the NICE guidance on 'Improving Outcomes in Urological Cancers', which was issued in 2002. The NICE guidance shows that national policy on PSA testing had relaxed slightly from a position of dissuasion to one focused even more on provision of information:

> One recent change to policy was the decision that PSA tests should be available to men who request them, but that they should first be provided with clear information about the test and the uncertainty about the balance of benefits and risks of screening for prostate cancer ... Patients should be offered material designed to promote informed choice about PSA tests.

The NICE guidance refers to the national HTA programme findings on screening, and emphasises an individual case approach: 'If physical examination of the prostate (DRE) suggested abnormality, or if symptoms or test results suggested the possibility of prostate cancer, then the man should be referred to a specialist prostate assessment clinic' (NICE, 2002).

The self-care movement

The rise of 'self-care' as a government-promoted concept is important in this consideration of prostate cancer detection, as well as the case of coagulometers discussed in this book. Although there is debate about the value of expert patient programmes (Kennedy et al., 2003), the discourse of self-care is becoming ubiquitous. As noted in the section above on usership, the availability of over-the-counter medical self-test kits is increasing and will continue to do so (POST, 2003). It is impossible to consider the PSA test entirely divorced from the context of ascertainment of the disease of prostate cancer itself and society's massive concerns with the treatment of cancers. Thus one of the many points of contention that the PSA test has become embroiled in is the question of 'awareness' of the disease. This issue erupts sporadically into the public sphere through the mass media, and awareness is frequently promoted as being a good thing, especially for men – typically portrayed as reluctant users of the healthcare system. Awareness of health issues is thus drawn in to the discourse of self-care. In the UK, the online and nurse-run advisory service NHS Direct poses on its website as a 'Common Health Question' 'Why aren't all men given a PSA test?', with the explanation emphasising the uncertainty of symptom development, the lack of evidence that screening would reduce mortality rates and the relatively poor technical performance of the test itself. Thus self-care in the context of PSA testing highlights the boundary between use and non-use of the technology.

Risk management

The policy on PSA testing in Britain has been relatively conservative, as noted above, in an attempt to control diffusion of the practice to large sectors of the male population. The nation-wide HTA ProtecT study, referred to in parliamentary answers and mentioned above in the sections on science and cancer screening, forms part of a wider NHS Prostate Cancer Programme, in turn part of the policy initiative known as the NHS Plan launched by the Department of Health in 2000 (NHS Executive, 2000). The focus is the so-called PCRMP, officially launched in 2001, although applying only to England at the time. The science of HTA and risk management policy are explicitly combined here. The programme has several dimensions, primarily aiming at facilitating provision of information about testing to asymptomatic men in order for us to make 'informed choices' about proceeding with the test, measures to speed up access to diagnosis and treatment, and advice to GPs.

An expert advisory group was convened by the government's Department of Health, comprising leading representatives of GPs, radiologists, urological surgeons, oncologists, practice nurses, pathologists, a statistician, the Director of the African Diaspora Association and the director of the National Screening Committee (Watson et al., 2002). An information sheet was developed for men requesting a PSA test, formalising the model of informed choice. The National Cancer Director wrote to hospital pathology requirements expressing concern about the possibility of standardisation of test procedures:

> Given that approximately two thirds of men undergoing TRUS [transrectal ultrasound] biopsy because of an elevated PSA are not found to have cancer ... The best management for those with a persistently elevated PSA but negative biopsies is unclear. These men may face prolonged periods of follow up and experience considerable anxiety.
> (Watson et al, 2002)

In summary, public policy on the PSA test for prostate cancer is dominated by actions focused on issues of population-level effectiveness and iatrogenic healthcare risk, rather than technological safety. Over the last decade UK policy has been developed at the highest possible levels of regulation-informing science and of a public management regime institutionalised into the centralised healthcare state machinery.

Ironically, this scientific and political centralisation has served to construct and solidify the controversy and risk associated with the use of PSA technology, and to support a diffusion of knowledge of – and uncertainty about – the test among healthcare communities as well as broad sectors of society.

The dynamics of PSA test innovation and governance

This chapter tackles questions about the dynamics of PSA technology in several dimensions: relations between science and governance and clinical practice; risk, citizenship, usership and patienthood; and the development of HTA science.

The healthcare science (HTA) of the PSA test was moving into the era of regulatory evidentiality in the mid 1990s, and the PSA test–prostate cancer-screening issue became iconic. The new multidisciplinary healthcare sciences became enrolled in state-orchestrated policy legitimation structures. Arguably, the high degree of public and political controversy associated with PSA played an important role in embedding HTA and the concept of scientific evidence-based healthcare into emerging governance institutions.

In the context of a policy *not* to introduce a public screening programme, it is clear that at the beginning of the twenty-first century there is considerable ambiguity in existing policies and practices, and confusion among both the medical profession and men concerned about the disease. Men with urinary problems in the UK are likely to be PSA-tested either by GPs or by NHS urologists, and may be tested by insurance-funded private medical companies (even without their knowledge). The urological profession, healthcare scientists and governmental trends have combined to elevate the degree of information provision to men and magnify the health service incursion into asymptomatic men's appraisal of personal risk and healthcare decisions. Screening in the UK may have been creeping in through the back door (Donovan et al., 2001) – exactly what policymakers have been seeking to avoid. One implication of this is that more men than is justified by the existing science will have been exposed to further investigation and to radical treatment. This is supported by the practice of medical practitioners motivated, especially, by high levels of concern about missing possible life-threatening diagnoses.

Societally negotiated standards about the degree of safety risk generated by the technical practice of PSA testing are inscribed into formal regulatory controls over entry to the marketplace and post-implementation surveillance of device technologies. The IVMDD regulation provides for a relatively high standard of evidence of the technical performance of PSA test equipment, although this remains the responsibility of the Notified Body system comprising private companies mandated by the 'competent authorities' of the EU-centralised regulatory system. Thus the high-risk designation of the PSA test builds into the technical requirements for PSA technology recognition of society's generally high concern about the consequences of detecting or not detecting cancer in the population.

There have been divisions within the medical and surgical professions on PSA over the last decade and this continues in professional debate over recent evidence, suggesting doubt about the value of the PSA test: 'Many urologists and other physicians have received the P.S.A. test, perhaps because they don't consider the issue of screening to be uncertain ... They believe the test works, but our results don't support that position' (*New York Times*, 10 January, 2006 'Report Casts Fresh Doubts On Prostate Cancer Testing'; cf. Concato et al., 2006).

As the discussion of men's experience of the PSA test shows, there is extreme ambivalence within the population about the value of the test and this is reflected to some extent in decisions to undergo it. The institutionalised HTA science and governmental representation of this science has constructed men as ambiguously confronted by 'informed choice' and 'shared' medical decision-making. Individual men can experience extreme ambivalence as a result of confronting the test. The extent of this uncertainty has been commented on by academic clinicians who have assessed the UK government's risk management programme for prostate cancer as embodying an 'institutional uncertainty' (Evans et al., 2007). The analysis presented here supports this insight.

The large, national HTA-supported ProtecT trial introduced innovative uses of qualitative methodology, and constructs a novel, uncertain, risky, evidential space which contains interaction between participating men and nurses and urologists. In these spaces, information about the uncertainties of PSA testing and prostate cancer treatment, and the meaning of aspects of healthcare science is conveyed to and discussed with men in a 'counselling' mode. This recalls, for example, interpretation of healthcare counselling practices in which distinctions between information and advice can be difficult to disentangle (Silverman, 1997). Thus the enrolment of members of the population into long-term knowledge-producing healthcare laboratories is accomplished through methodologies which attend to experience, anxiety, language use and choice-making. The scientific work is also framed as a participative methodology, in which 'users' may be seen as beneficiaries of the research process they themselves are contributing to.

In summary, innovation of the use of PSA technology into the health-care system can be characterised by two observations. Firstly, PSA innovation is at the centre of a nexus of conflicting forces of scientific knowledge, professional powers and citizen-patient variability, which is reflected and enhanced in a high level of governmental institutionalisation. Secondly, the dynamics of science and governance in this field have promoted societal knowledge and risk related to PSA while attempting to regulate the diffusion of the test itself among the population. This chapter has in effect charted the rise of the PSA test and the complicated status that it has achieved in contemporary healthcare and health experience. It will be interesting to follow its pathway in the future, now that the demise of the technology has been announced by the very clinical scientists who once enthusiastically introduced it (Stamey et al., 2004).

PSA technology and society

PSA testing for prostate cancer has penetrated the public domain of citizenship to a degree and in a way that the other technologies considered in this book have not. Arguably, it has become *more 'social'* than the other device technologies analysed here. Many of the controversies around this field have been highly emotive. Those arguing against the use of the PSA test in screening programmes, for example, have been accused of geriatricide.

Testing for prostate cancer has become, in crude terms, a victim of its own success – in a way similar to the success of hip replacement technology in the case study in this book. Unlike, for example, artificial hips, the PSA technology is even less stabilised in the collective practices of healthcare and policy, reflecting its acknowledged low level of functional performance. While there is some development of variants to the basic technology, these are of limited significance in the sociomedical sphere because of the extreme salience of the interpretive practices in the usership of the test, both as a collective medical practice and in the consumption of the test by citizens/patients.

The PSA test is a technology that cannot be considered from society's point of view without also considering widely shared meanings of cancer and assumptions about diagnostic tests, which have built up over several decades as part of cultural and healthcare visions, and which as the development of the PSA test and other tests show, are far from immutable.

Indeed, it is likely that the very concept of a medical diagnostic test and the social, organisational and medical culture surrounding the ordering of medical tests for citizens is already being changed under the pressure of technological developments, especially in the field of genetics.

The technical science of performance *per se* plays a lesser part in this technology, while health*care* science is very prominent. The national healthcare state plays a prominent role in shaping the trajectory of the technology. In the UK both national HTA science and coordinated medical professional activity have interacted with the state, with the effect of amplifying knowledge of the scientific uncertainty of PSA practice. This has been consolidated through the creation of dedicated political regulatory activity and institutions in the UK such as the national risk management programme. The state's aims, however, achieved limited success. Regulatory policy is countered by various forces that have been described.

The most salient evidence in the field of PSA testing is the *lack* of definitive or even suggestive evidence about the value of the test as a detection technology. Indeed, there are clearly conflicting constructions of what the appropriate evidence is with which society might understand and respond to the dilemmas of PSA. In this situation the socio-scientific-medical space that the various stakeholders might inhabit is magnified and has become a scientifically complex and existentially worrying zone. This uncertainty extends to the evidence presented in this chapter – for example, the striking disjuncture between personal testimonials of men's experience of the PSA test and that derived from the application of 'quality of life' measurement tools by clinical and healthcare scientists.

An effect akin to medicalisation has been occurring in the case of PSA – the technology has become widely diffused and the medical practices associated with it have been promoted outside the clinic – but this is not straightforward linear medicalisation. It is, rather, a medicalisation that configures men as to-be-counselled patients and as citizens placed in the position of having to make 'informed choices' about exposing themselves to the technology or not. Here, medicalisation paradoxically carries its own scientific uncertainty into society as a diffusion of risk perceptions. Thus the parameters of the 'laboratory of the NHS' (Faulkner, 1997) are extended. Given the widely diverging individual responses to the technology, on the one hand some men behave as the informed choice-makers that governance, science and medical professions have constructed, but, equally, some men have experienced their encounter with the technology in terms of victimhood rather than active citizenship.

Usership of PSA testing has been constructed as an activity of informed interpretation. Science and governance have combined to define a counselling-based model of information-giving, which echoes the move towards shared decision-making that is to be found in other fields of medical practice. In scientific studies of PSA there have been forged a hybrid sociomedical space, constituting an engagement between science and society that combines elements of the scientific enterprise and pastoral care. It is worth recalling here that Foucault deemed pastoral care to be 'the premier technique of power in late modern societies' (Foucault, 1981, cited in Bloor, 2001). This negotiated form of engagement is legitimised by being designed into national, government-backed science and policy agendas and contained in the public policy buffer zones of healthcare science. Through this novel socio-scientific space, healthcare science can be constituted as 'user-friendly', and healthcare governance can be constituted as managing policymakers' and individual risks and fears, and clinicians' scientific uncertainty. The state, in its political intervention and in its enrolment of healthcare science, has developed a position of custodianship here. Unlike the traditional model of the paternalism of the medical profession, however, this custodianship does not operate via claims to cognitive authority but via carefully designed invitations to the sharing of uncertainty and risk.

While the concept of interpretative flexibility has been used in Social Construction of Technology studies to account for the development of technologies along different design pathways (as, for example, in bicycle design – Bijker, 1995), here it can be applied also to the societal use of a technology. The lesser visibility of the material technology itself means that proliferation of different types and variants of the PSA test has not become a major policy issue, unlike, for example, artificial hips and infusion pumps. Indeed, the state policy here supports proliferation as it forms part of the search for better-performing testing technology.

In conclusion, the evidence and analysis presented in this chapter indicate that the PSA pathway in healthcare has been defined by national-level scientific production of uncertainty about the societal value of the technology and the risks of its use for cancer detection. Multi-stakeholder governance institutions have been created on this foundation, which, in turn, have diffused science-legitimated uncertainties to citizens while attempting to contain uninformed diffusion of PSA practice. Thus, the PSA case could be summarised as one in which scientifically assessed *risk* has constructed *governance* – which in turn has constructed a social sharing of risk.

6

Infusion Pumps: Usership and the Governance of Error

with Mara Clécia Dantas Souza

Introduction

The 'drip' standing beside the bed of hospital patients is one of the most common public images of intensive hospital care. Indeed it is one of the most ubiquitous devices in technological healthcare. Contemporary infusion pumps are devices that deliver medicinal fluids, nutrition, blood and blood products. The technology comprising and controlling the drip is extremely diverse, ranging from the relatively simple to the very complex. Guided by an electromechanical pump, infusions can be delivered to the human body with high and controlled pressures to provide regulated amounts of fluids intravenously, or epidurally (just within the surface of the central nervous system). The process can be prolonged over periods of time that would be impossible to maintain in everyday healthcare practice. The technology typically comprises mechanical, electrical, electronic and software components. Fixed and ambulatory applications are found. Some infusion devices are implantable, though these are not considered in this chapter.

In the UK's NHS over seven million infusions are delivered to patients annually. The healthcare situations and settings in which infusion pumps are used vary very widely, including critical care and high-dependency, palliative care and neonatal intensive care. The devices are typically operated by nurses, and other health professionals including anaesthetists and clinicians may also operate them at the bedside. They are regarded as labour-saving devices. This technology is implicated in emotive life situations including pain relief for patients with cancer, other life-threatening conditions and in some countries, assisted suicide.

Some of the world's largest medical device companies produce and distribute infusion pumps. The complexity of the marketplace for infusion pumps and the complexity of individual devices is evident both in the number of features designed into them and the wide range that may be deployed in healthcare settings.

The benefits brought by the large-scale application of this form of therapeutic provision are indisputable. The contemporary complex intravenous (IV) drug therapies would be impossible without the infusion pump. However, there are a number of risks associated with infusion pump technology and their use in healthcare practice. Manufacture and design problems and mistakes in use do occur, and the healthcare system is struggling with the boundary between these two types of risk. According to data from the UK's MHRA, infusion devices are second only to implantable devices in their association with fatalities (Dunn et al., 2006). The performance of infusion pumps in hospital practice has become an issue of increasing concern for healthcare policymakers and regulators internationally over the last 10–15 years. They have attracted an increasingly high level of attention from regulatory authorities, and many healthcare policymakers, monitoring agencies and hospital/clinical managers have placed the technology high on their agendas for improvement. Alleged problems arise in many areas – organisational, human resource and expertise, design and engineering technology, workplace and job design and the nature of the commercial marketplace and its interface with healthcare systems. As will become clear in this chapter, a concern about infusion pumps and IV therapy is closely tied to the promotion of 'patient safety' as part of the core agenda among healthcare policymaking communities.

Infusion pumps as a material technology make a useful case study for this book because of the complexity of the components and especially the dependence on skilled programming by users in nursing and therapeutic working environments. In addition, there is an intimate linkage of use of the technology to critical clinical decision-making, organisational communication and hospital information systems. This chapter draws upon a variety of documentary and primary research sources, especially the work of co-author Mara Souza, who conducted participatory fieldwork and interviews with medical device regulatory agencies in the UK during 2005–6, having previously undertaken extensive primary research on the electromedical device healthcare and regulatory system in Brazil.[1]

Epidemiology and the marketplace

It is difficult to assess with any accuracy the epidemiology of diseases and medical conditions for which infusion pumps might be deployed because of the many clinical conditions and functions for which they are used. They may be used in critical care, high-dependency care, palliative care, surgery, paediatric care, oncology, haematology and neonatal care.

Their primary uses are for the delivery of pharmaceutical agents to alleviate pain, for delivering blood and blood products and nutrition. 'Parenteral' nutrition – intravenous feeding – is widely practiced for patients who cannot swallow or digest foodstuff. Some chemotherapy drugs for cancer therapy are delivered manually by syringe, but where a controlled infusion is required it is known that dosing is often administered too rapidly, a problem frequently attributed to staffing pressures in the organisation. Thus pump-driven syringes are attractive as a technological aid in these circumstances.

Patients in critical care often require long-term IV administrations of potent drugs which have very small margins for error. Unfortunately, errors in the delivery of medication occur at relatively high rates in all healthcare systems, and this is a major factor influencing the designers and developers of infusion devices. Adverse drug events are the single major cause of all medical injuries, so there is a strong incentive to develop technology-aided approaches to reducing errors. The interplay of a discourse of technical rationality with other frames in which the delivery of medication is construed as a problem is one of the main themes to be analysed in this chapter.

Infusion pumps are part of the medical equipment sector which is highly globalised. In terms of the number of devices distributed across the world, it is estimated, for example, that one of the most widely used infusion pumps produced by Baxter International in the mid-2000s had 152,260 devices distributed in 25 countries, including the UK (Food and Drug Administration, 2005). One of the Alaris Medical Systems products had 55,200 devices in use in the US and Canada (Food and Drug Administration, 2004). The major infusion pumps companies operating and distributing devices in the UK are: Abbot, Arcomedical, Baxter International, B. Braun, Cardinal Health, Codan, Fresenius, Medtronic, Nutricia, Roche and Smiths Medical (MHRA, 2006). The largest company is Baxter International, which supplies nearly every hospital in the UK with medical equipment of some sort; equipment for delivery of medication is one of their primary activities.

Development of infusion pump technology

An external infusion pump was first described in 1945 (Dickenson, 1983 cited in Graham & Clark, 2005). Syringe drivers to provide controlled infusion were developed in the 1950s in the UK and were adopted from an original haematology application into palliative care. This has become a commonly used technique in palliative care in the UK. In the 1960s, electrical power was added in some designs to the 1950s' basic plunger-timer concept. Invention of the volumetric (non-syringe) electromedical infusion pump has been credited to a Dr. Hess, at B. Braun company, in 1951, in Germany (Invest in Germany GMBH, 2005; Dunn, 2006). The first *programmable* infusion devices, introduced in the late 1960s, were single-channel devices limited to relatively simple rate and volume programming.

A general infusion system is made of three elements: a reservoir for containing material in fluid form, a catheter and a control device which powers and regulates the flow of liquid. The aim is to achieve very precise, pre-set control over the delivery of the fluid material. If pumps are not available in a care setting, or if changes in the flow rate would not have serious clinical consequences for the recipient, a 'gravity drip' may otherwise be used. Electromedical infusion pumps are 'active controller' devices.

There are different classifications of pumps. Large volumetric pumps are produced for 'medium and high flow rate and large volume infusions' (MDA, 2003) such as pumping nutrient solutions to feed a patient. These operate either by a peristaltic mechanism or with cassette mechanisms. Smaller-volume pumps infuse pharmaceuticals such as hormones, for example insulin in cases of diabetes, or opiates. Syringe infusion pumps are preferred for lower volume and low rate infusion (MDA, 2003). These classifications are important because of the different clinical applications involved, which imply different regulatory and work-setting regimes. Despite similar intended uses, infusion pumps can have very different design, material and working principles, and manufacturers continually produce innovations.

From an engineering point of view, contemporary infusion pumps are based on electro-electronics and mechanical-material technology. Recent refinements of the systems have been made especially in the introduction of software and IT communication features. Contemporary pumps typically have a range of in-built safety features, including protection against 'single failure' (a failure that triggers an alarm), alarms, log files of activity, pre-programming for medicines and, very recently, bar-code technology for linking specific medicines to specific patients with specific clinical requirements.

Onboard software is an important part of contemporary systems and can be provided, for example, for programmed dose-control. This can help the operator to calculate the infusion rate, can identify medicines from a database and preset the maximum and minimum volume or rate for a specific patient. One of the major trends in the development of infusion pump technology is the development of linkages to other systems via communications technology. If the healthcare service has a compatible IT system, the software in the pump can be programmed to identify the patient in hospital information systems and notify the operator if a dose prescribed is outside the standard parameters set. Internal data logging functions can record all programming done by the operator or operators. Due to the major health risks and safety concerns associated with the pumps (explored in detail in the section below on governance), manufacturers increasingly highlight safety features, especially to reduce dosing errors. 'Smart' pumps are infusion systems that allow the entry of drug infusion rules (protocols) into a 'library' that can then be used to specify pre-defined limits to doses to be administered. As an example, the design and implementation of one such system at Harvard University/Massachusetts General Hospital has been described (Kinnealey et al., 2003). Audible alarms indicate if dose limits have been exceeded. For example, the company that claims to have introduced the first 'smart' pump, Cardinal Health in the US, makes the following claim about its latest developments:

> The Alaris® System with Guardrails® Suite of safety software ... combines dose error reduction software, a bedside computer, ... as well as continuous respiratory monitoring and bar code identification capabilities onto a single platform. Wireless connectivity capabilities also enable clinicians to transmit data automatically ... to existing clinical information systems and electronic patient records ... Managing multiple infusion pumps on the ward can be demanding ... To simplify your workflow, we offer a centralised fluid management system that allows ... automatically gathering data from each pump.
> (Cardinal Health, 2007)

The use of such 'smart' infusion devices and networking of infusion pump systems is widely recommended to reduce medication adminis-tration errors (Taxis, 2005).[2] The larger manufacturers generally have introduced such features. Manufacturers have claimed that smart pumps can avert one potentially life threatening error every 2.6 days at an aver-age 350-bed hospital (Husch et al., 2005). However, some doubts have been raised about the effectiveness of such systems in the working envi-ronment (see 'The sciences of usership' section below, and Taxis, 2005).

Such pumps may be developed with a view to their operability and *credibility* in the local context in which they will be deployed:

> provides our clinicians with a dynamic, less-complex system of safe drug delivery via an institutionally defined, clinician developed, hospital-sanctioned, customizable electronically loadable drug 'library' for all IV drugs that is housed in the infusion pump residing at the bedside.
>
> (Kinnealey et al., 2003)

The reference here to a system that is configured, customised and accepted in the local context is significant as an attempt to take into account users' and purchasers' antipathy towards 'one size fits all' technologies.

Since they were launched commercially, therefore, infusion pumps have grown greatly in technical complexity (Lefever, 2006). In the 1980s, the controls and features in most infusion pumps could be summarised as being to set the infusion rate, stop/start switch and alarms for power failure and the end of infusion or occlusion incidents. Contemporary pumps reportedly can have 62 alarms or warnings, 21 ways of setting the delivery rate or volume, 12 different settings for end of infusion point and six different nurse call-back alarm tones (Lefever, 2006).

Regulatory divergence: varieties of safety and performance

Infusion pump technology has become the object of a wide variety of regulatory activity globally. This activity includes the application of pre-existing technical standards, for example for electrical safety, the application of conformity assessment procedures under the EU MDD, and the creation of *de novo* reporting metrics and usability assessments.

Infusion pumps are classed as risk category II-b under the prevailing interpretation of the MDD in the EU, in other words the second-highest ('medium-high') level of risk. This requires third-party scrutiny under the terms of the devolved regime for certification of new devices to place them on the market. In this section, we point to a well recognised lacuna in the coverage of standards and regulation of medical devices, which is particularly important for understanding the modes of governance around infusion pumps that have emerged over the last decade.

International standards for medical electrical equipment have existed since the late 1960s and early 1970s, organised by the International Electrotechnical Commission (IEC). Their coverage has included manufacture, installation and application of electromedical equipment and its impact on patients and users. The main standard is expressed in a long series of documents that focus mainly on 'safety' aspects. On the other hand, the MDD of the 1990s were primarily geared towards objectives of free trade within Europe. The technical standards are much more detailed than the 'essential requirements' of the device directives. As a representative of an NHS Trust hospital in the UK explained:

> the essential requirements (of the Directive) have got ... a very short bit in there about electrical safety but there is a huge raft of standards that deal with the safety of electro-medical equipment and if you're designing a piece of electro-medical equipment and you want to place it on the market and you use the right safety standard then you can put a tick in the box against meeting the essential requirement on electrical safety.
>
> (interview, Hospital Clinical Engineer, 2006)

However, this construction of what constitutes safety differs from other metrics by which electromedical equipment such as infusion pumps might be evaluated. Alongside (electrical) safety, regulatory actors also use the concept of 'performance' to construe the assessment of devices:

> the standards are helpful in providing a ... basic, basic protection on safety, now in providing the best possible healthcare you perhaps also want performance criteria ... how the device can best achieve the therapeutic performance, because in many situations you may have something which is safe ... one is about absolute safety, causing no harm, the other is about ways of getting optimal health benefit and there is a gap between the two.
>
> (interview, NHS PASA Centre for
> Evidence-based Purchasing official, 2006)

Thus the performance in practice of equipment such as infusion pumps is elusive, and is not, perhaps cannot, be comprehensively defined by tests for performance criteria such as efficacy or effectiveness in clinical practice. It is in this area of uncertainty and flexibility in the legislative regulatory regime that the effects of usership come into the frame. Thus, in spite of the applicability of international electrical equipment standards to infusion pumps, there are no formal or informal standards for the design of infusion pump user *interfaces*. In 2003 the MHRA reported an analysis of 1495 incidents of which the cause in 53 per cent was unknown, 23 per cent were attributed to the device and 27 per cent to 'user error'; the implication being that much of the unknown 53 per cent was likely to be attributed to human error. Another official from the PASA, reflecting on the regime as it applied in practice to infusion pumps, made the ambiguity of usership explicit when he stated that:

> I think all the pumps are pretty much up to scratch in terms of accuracy, but some of them are very difficult to use (...). It's not always echoed in what happens unfortunately, so there will be an investigation and the finding is user-error. Some nurses get fired which is not either a solution and unfair. The standards are beginning to recognise that.
>
> (Interview, NHS PASA Centre for Evidence-based Purchasing official, 2006)

This regulatory actor is indicating that the way in which the official analysis of infusion pump safety risks is constructed, and the resulting allocation of responsibility for 'error', may have been biased towards user error and may be insufficiently sensitive to designs which make for usability problems.

There are, therefore, divergences in the ways in which infusion (and other) devices are evaluated and these are embedded in institutionalised regulatory regimes. There is what we might call an acknowledged 'evaluation gap' in the safety-related usership of infusion pumps. As this chapter will show, the existence of this gap between evaluatory boundaries leads to uncertainties between governance agencies attempting to understand and combat perceived problems with the technology.

Usership, practice and error

Nurses and medical practitioners such as anaesthetists are the main *clinical* users of infusion pumps. They are also frequently worked with by pharmacists and by biomedical engineers or clinical engineers for medication standards and control, programming, customisation and maintenance activities. Thus interaction with infusion pumps occurs in a variety of healthcare work roles, requiring different types of knowledge, expertise and competencies. A single NHS Trust in the UK may have several hundred infusion pumps installed, and a similar level of diffusion of the devices can be found elsewhere.

Notice of the results of the use of infusion pumps percolate into the public domain from time to time, sometimes in the wake of tragic events:

> A jury inquest in March last year determined Mr X had been unlawfully killed after receiving 10 times the normal dosage of painkillers … Magistrates heard an infusion pump had been wrongly set after a simple mathematical miscalculation had been made by a consultant anaesthetist (who) … admitted after this tragic human case to not being experienced in the use of the specific infusion pump.
>
> (*Llanelli Star*, March 15, 2001)

Reports such as this from Wales, UK, raise obvious issues for policymakers and health service managers about the specialisation of particular models of the technology, specialist training and expertise, communication within the hospital organisation and legal liabilities. The example serves to highlight the way in which risks associated with this technology are represented in the public domain, which undoubtedly have influenced policymaking communities' apprehension of infusion and medication-related error. The policy and governance developments relevant to these devices are discussed in more detail below.

The types of competence and expertise that are invoked by infusion pumps for their operators include nursing and medical knowledge, knowledge of administration of medicines, product selection, manual abilities such as assembling components and the 'sets' that contain the material to be administered, mathematical and calculative skills and skills in digital programming. More generally required are competencies in working in a complex sociomedical technological environment, responding appropriately to audible alarms and working with a range of non-standardised human interfaces in the same workplace. Such skills generally require training, and such training may be at least to some degree specific to particular pump designs or families. The issue of user-ship skills and training raises questions that are at the heart of policymakers' and regulators' concerns with contemporary infusion pump–related healthcare delivery.

The different scientific, regulatory, policymaker and professional user stakeholders in the field of IV infusion conceive and construct the issues of infusion pump performance in different ways with different emphases. In order to understand the multidimensional usership of these devices, it is necessary first to present a more detailed description of the range of functions comprised by infusion devices. This will enable what we might call the social construction of error in this field to be highlighted. Users of infusion pumps may act in a variety of ways to determine the configuration of pumps and related technology that is implemented. We can distinguish between purchasing decisions and subsequent implementation decisions that set up an infusion pump system in a hospital or other healthcare setting.

Constructing understandings of error

There are many types of failure reported in the UK and internationally with infusion pumps. These include programming errors, infection, electromagnetic interference, mechanical malfunction and 'human error' (see Table 6.1). It is clear that the construction of what constitutes 'error' is contested in the case of infusion pumps. Different disciplines, different regulatory agencies, industrial actors and healthcare strategists are involved in varying and sometimes conflicting attempts to define error and assess causes and accountabilities.

Many studies have been conducted to assess the prevalence of medication errors. In the US, Husch et al. (2005) used epidemiological methods (preferred to less reliable information from incident report-ing databases). Their study observed prospectively that in 286 patients receiving infusion therapy in 426 medication deliveries, almost 70 per cent of IV doses were associated with at least one error of some sort, including three (out of 389) errors potentially causing temporary harm or prolonging hospitalisation. Other studies have shown IV error rates varying between 27 and 49 per cent (Wirtz et al., 2003). An ethnographic study in 2003 in the *British Medical Journal* suggested that in the UK medication errors occurred with 49 per cent of all IV medications administered, 73 per cent of these errors

Table 6.1 Regulatory agency analysis of 1495 infusion pump incidents

Cause of incident	Percent of incidents (n=1495)
Damage (dropping the device, etc); miss settings/tampering	4%
Faulty quality assurance systems	4%
Software issues	5%
Electrical/mechanical issues	7%
Maintenance issues	7%
The design of the device	8%
User error	19%
Unknown cause	46%

Source: (adapted from MHRA, 2003)

occurred with pumped medications and 95 per cent of those occurred when nurses administered doses faster than recommended (Taxis and Barber, 2003).

The hospital working environment for nurses in particular may be extremely complex (see Figure 6.1). Apart from a wide variety of patients, technologies and pharmaceutical preparations, infusion equipment and monitoring devices typically have built-in audible alarms, which may be triggered by many different events. One American study was reported to have found that in a period of 298 hours in one hospital ward area there were 325 alarms silenced, more than 90 per cent of which were false (Tsien and Fackler, 2004, cited by Davidson & Barber, 2004). The UK's MHRA produced the following classification of causes for incidents reported over a five-year period.

The large percentage of unclassified causes illustrates the difficulty that official agencies have experienced in identifying causes of incidents. The complexity of establishing 'root causes' can be illustrated by examining a list of problems listed in a formal alert issued by the MHRA on one model of infusion device. These include, for example, gearbox

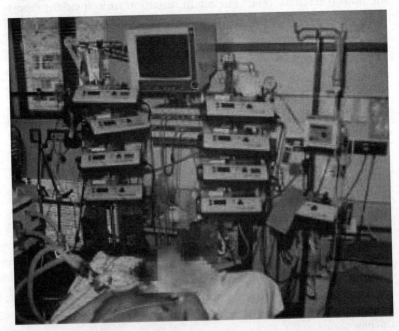

Figure 6.1 Infusion pumps may be part of a complex working environment requiring a wide variety of expertise

Table 6.2 Types of user error identified by the UK regulatory agency for devices

Misloading the giving set or syringe
Setting the wrong rate
Confusing primary and secondary rates
Not confirming the set rate
Not confirming the pump type or syringe size
Not stopping the pump correctly
Allowing free-flow when lines are changed
Unskilled or irregular servicing
Inadequate testing after servicing
Interference by patients or visitors

wear, false air-in-line alarms, under-infusion caused by misloaded infusion sets and undercharged battery. Such problems clearly include a mixture of 'technological' and 'social' aspects.

Given that alleged user error is large, a report from the MHRA has listed a wide range of typical types of such error that occur with the use if infusion pumps (MDA, 2003), as given in Table 6.2.

The question of how user error may be defined by different stakeholders is raised acutely by this type of representation of infusion pump performance. Note that in this classification the users identified may be patients, visitors or engineers as well as nursing and other clinical personnel. As will be seen in the following sections, there has been a general shift during the last decade away from a discourse of *user* error towards a less blaming, more organisation-oriented official classification of '*use* error'.

The sciences of usership

We have pointed out the central importance of the ambivalent concepts of performance and usership in recent developments in the growth of the assessment of processes of innovation of the technology into the healthcare system. A range of scientific approaches are being brought to bear on infusion pump performance that have implications both for feedback into technological design and for the management of gatekeeping processes affecting adoption. Scientific studies pertinent to this field range from engineering performance and usability testing to developments in the methodology of investigating performance and 'failures' and their causes. In this section, we present some illustrations of these sciences applied to the usership of infusion devices.

A conspicuous scientific approach to technology–human interfaces is ergonomics, associated with a 'human factors' approach to usability testing. This discipline has turned its attention to infusion pump performance. The human factors approach, widely used in engineering and organisation analysis, arguably employs an individualised model of usership. It may comprise '(1) observations of use and interviews with users in order to map the environmental context and tasks, (2) a critical evaluation of the infusion pump by heuristic evaluation and a cognitive walk-through of its interface, (3) an analysis of reported incidents, and (4) applying theory about mental capacity and human error' (Garmer et al., 2002).

Echoing the classification produced by the MHRA (Table 6.2), the sorts of errors that were identified in a single study included 'pushing the wrong button' for example, pressing button for volume-to-be-infused (VTBI) when actually trying to read off the volume already delivered; entering the wrong value for the flow rate; confusing the VTBI and rate of flow to be set and entering the wrong VTBI. Subjective assessments by users included ease of correcting errors, confidence in having set the infusion correctly, speed of operation and learning and need to refer to a manual. The same study suggested that nurse-users may be the source of suggestions for design improvements. Examples of suggestions were: 'avoid several functions on the same button' and 'confirmation that setting has been completed' (adapted from Garmer et al., 2002). These authors noted that in tests users were often able to notice their own errors and rectify them, concluding that this suggests a requirement that interfaces be 'self-instructional' and for a high level of 'guessability' – a quality that was low in both device interfaces that were tested in the study.[3]

Garmer et al. conclude with the suggestion, interesting in terms of sociological understanding of the extent to which technology is a designer-based 'black-box' or modifiable through learning processes and user participation (cf. Hyysalo, 2004; Stewart and Williams, 2005):

> This study further indicates that the users of medical equipment might need to be actively supported and trained to question design solutions otherwise user problems might not be highlighted in the development phase.

Similar ergonomic analysis is part of the evaluations conducted by the UK's national Device Evaluation Centre for infusion pumps. Such evaluations examine a range of technical performance and usership/ usability issues (CEP, October 2007). In this evaluation, nurse users in a chemotherapy suite were positive about clarity of visual display, ease of inserting the infusion sets and the ability to operate two separate infusions simultaneously to the patient, but negative about a range of features including alarm loudness, text size, screen too busy, alarm difficult to interpret and slow keyboard entry (CEP, 2007).

The recent development of smart pumps has also been investigated in terms of performance and error. An evaluation in the journal *Quality and Safety in Health Care* suggests that the industry-generated claims for this technology should be carefully appraised (Taxis, 2005), referring to an analysis which, in contrast to common assumptions, estimated that only one out of 389 errors may have been prevented by smart pumps (Husch et al., 2005). This was largely because the pumps available are insufficiently integrated into other information systems. For example, they were not linked to an electronic prescribing system nor barcoded medicines administration. Taxis concluded that further development is required to be able to increase patient safety (Taxis, 2005). Referring to the UK's NPSA (2004b) pilot project (see below), and even aside from deficiencies in training and the wide range of different pumps in use, Taxis notes that

the software of devices of the same type had multiple configurations and therefore reacted differently under the same circumstances.

In a well-conducted study, rate errors due to misprogramming of the device by the user were 'surprisingly' rare, and the authors concluded that a tendency to equate infusion medication errors with programming errors is suspect. More common were 'latent' errors such as mislabelled infusion bags, misidentified patients and mismatch between the rate of infusion noted as ordered by the clinician and that labelled on the device. This research concluded that a major source of error lies in the organisational practicalities and systems of communication and response to clinical decisions, rather than in the user interface itself (Husch et al., 2005).

The second strand of scientific study of usership is more focused on analysis of error via different technical methodologies. A range of different methodologies are under development or are being adapted for application to understanding of risk and safety matters in healthcare in general and to medication administration in particular. A European funded project – the SIMPATIE Programme – supported by European Commission DG Health & Consumer Protection has surveyed and collected a range of different new and emerging methodologies for improving patient safety (http://www.simpatie.org). These included 'safety culture assessment' tools with techniques such as Healthcare Failure Mode and Effects

Analysis (HFMEA), and Root Cause Analysis. These two techniques are both starting to be used in the case of infusion pumps in the UK.

Failure Mode and Effects Analysis (FMEA) is an industrial tool developed by reliability engineers to evaluate complex processes, identify elements that have a risk, and prioritise remedies. The method uses information from a variety of sources to develop a scoring system and to predict the behaviour of a system in which failure might occur (Apkon et al., 2004). Thus this approach is likely to result in a questioning of understandings of error that highlight users of a technology and 'mistakes' that disattend the complexity of technological environments and sociomedical organisation:

> the frequency of failure, the complexity of the drug delivery process, and the number of individuals participating in the process suggest that it is more appropriate to consider medication errors to be failures of a drug *delivery system*.
>
> (Apkon et al., op. cit.)

This type of analysis is likely to construct complex models of different types of system failure including organisational, expertise, interface and technological elements (Fechter and Barba, 2004).

Both ergonomics and 'failure mode' analysis, therefore, can lead to a broadening of the terms in which errors in device performance are framed. The ergonomics focus on the user-device interface shows that users *interact* with devices and have the ability to develop and bring a range of competencies to bear on their work with the technology, including shaping of certain features of its design. Failure mode analysis, in particular, promotes a less user-oriented framing of error, which directs attention towards the socio-technological features of systems. Such alternative formulations of safety-related error are key to the development of policy and the regulation of infusion pump performance to which we now turn.

Policy and governance

Many surveillance and governance initiatives have been undertaken worldwide to try to understand and reduce the problems attributed to or associated with infusion pumps in healthcare practice. In the section above on 'Regulatory divergence' we noted how legislative definitions and jurisdictions create tensions in the institutional assessment of 'performance', with different agencies construing this in different ways, and with the possibility that important aspects of safety might be unclaimed under the statutory regulatory system. Our discussion of *usership science* highlighted some methodologies and disciplines that have moved to fill the gap in regulatory evaluation. We now turn to discuss how this focus on usership and usability has become related to the development of *'patient safety'* as a policy movement, and how this has been formulated in relation to infusion pump technology by those regulatory agencies involved.

Framing patient safety

A powerful policy agenda focused on 'patient safety' grew in importance during the 1990s in the UK, as elsewhere. In the UK it was strongly linked to the promotion of the clinical governance approach to organisational accountability. It was marked by the appearance of dedicated academic medical journals such as *Quality and Safety in Health Care*, published by the key *British Medical Journal* publishing group, and by the publication of major government reports which developed theories, frameworks and practice guidance for dealing with adverse incidents and for developing risk management in the healthcare system. In the UK the landmark policy work that set the policy direction was *An Organisation with a Memory* (Department of Health Expert Group, 2000). This report highlighted a lack of research into reporting and information systems for errors, incidents and device failures. A pilot study of hospitalised patients in London concluded that around 10 per cent of all inpatient episodes resulted in harmful adverse events, of which about half appeared preventable. The analysis distinguished between 'human error' and 'systemic effects', and emphasised a need for 'safety systems' and open organisational culture rather than blame culture. Safety systems in use in industry, especially the aviation industry, were assessed for their relevance to healthcare.

Also in the early 2000s, the UK Department of Health has made the subject of medication safety into a priority for *'Building a safer NHS'* (Department of Health, 2004). Again, this policy initiative identified IV infusion – among many other causes of medication problems – as requiring special attention. In addition, a specific research and policy agenda developed internationally during the early 2000s focused on the use of medicines for children. The development of scientific, regulatory and political action in medication and paediatric medication in particular has thus dovetailed with the framing of policy around patient safety, giving the focus on medication delivery heightened priority.

A National Patient Safety Agency in the UK

This policy movement led directly to the setting up in the UK of an agency dedicated to patient safety matters, the NPSA. A National Reporting and Learning System (NRLS) was created under the coordination of NPSA to provide a single point for reporting patient safety incidents involving NHS patients. The system classifies different types of incidents and was planned to be incorporated into hospital risk management software. At the heart of the NPSA's remit to gather and analyse incident data systematically is the modernist methodology of 'root cause analysis', as noted above: the UK Parliamentary Under-Secretary of State for Health defined it as: 'A structured investigation that aims to investigate the true cause of a problem and the actions necessary to eliminate it ... it is about drilling down into the underlying management and organisational factors' (Emslie et al., 2002). In this and a series of recent national policy documents such as *Doing Less Harm* and *Building a safer NHS for patients* much is made of a need to establish the systemic causes of adverse incidents. *Safety first* (Department of Health et al.; 2006) further extended both national central safety-oriented forums and local healthcare organisations for implementation of safety initiatives. Infusion pumps as medication delivery technologies are frequently highlighted in these agenda-defining accounts of safety issues.

A range of regulatory agencies and government groups have become involved in issues of adoption and diffusion on infusion pump technology in the UK. On the government side, the NAO indicated the growing significance of a patient safety agenda in 2005 (NAO, 2005; Figure 6.2), and in the same year an All-Party Parliamentary Group for Patient Safety was established. As will be evident below, technology appraisal and healthcare guidance agency NICE is conspicuously absent from this account.

Regulating infusion pump performance

Infusion pumps were one of the technologies that figured large in the international conference that launched the NPSA:

> If most of us cannot programme our video recorder timer then why would you expect us to be able to programme a modern infusion pump?
>
> (Barach, 2002)

We can note here the rhetorical parallel drawn with video recorder programming – a highlighting of a 'user expertise' frame of reference which, as we noted above, (Constructing understandings of error)

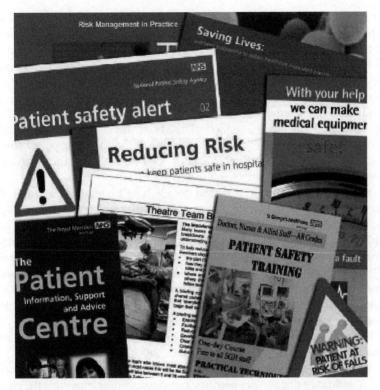

Figure 6.2 The cover of the UK National Audit Office report *A Safer Place for Patients*

should not be taken at face value. Drawing 'lessons from Australia' at the same launch meeting, Runciman provided an analysis of the high level of Heparin (for peri-operative blood-thinning) incidents nationally. This showed that

> the culprits are miscalculation of doses for infusion and misuse of infusion pumps ... 60% of the problems were ultimately caused by the lack of standardisation of the makes and models of infusion pumps.
>
> (Runciman, 2002)

Again, an issue of usership skills is foregrounded. In the same iconic conference, Pickstone emphasised the complexity of IV medication risks. Drawing on the field of industrial accidents, an 'infusion pump driving test' approach to improvement had been developed (Pickstone and Quinn, 2002). In an analysis of one NHS hospital's infusion related practices in the 1990s, Quinn presented a picture of multiple models of technology, lack of purchasing strategy, unused and hoarded equipment, a high proportion of obsolete equipment and lack of training. These leading activists in infusion device safety analysis and management reported success with standardising pump purchasing, stock-keeping and training schemes for 'proper use' (Pickstone and Quinn, 2002), which reportedly led to a reduction in adverse incidents in the hospital in question. Patient safety, therefore, is one of the emerging policy contexts in which the concerted focus on IV drug delivery and infusion pumps has become strongly framed.

Regulatory agencies over the last decade have increasingly attempted to assess the scope of problems associated with the safety and usership of infusion pumps in healthcare systems around the world. Much of this effort has been made in recognition of a dearth of systematic information previously accessible. In Brazil, for example, the National Health Surveillance Agency (ANVISA) published a Technovigilance Information Bulletin on the subject (ANVISA, 2004). During the 2006 Global Harmonisation Task Force Conference, speakers from worldwide regulatory agencies highlighted infusion pumps as a prime example of risky equipment, special reference being made to deficiencies in usability (participant observation by MS, 28–30 June 2006, Lübeck).

In the UK, in 2000 and again in 2002, the MDA had published 'one-liner' guidance documents pointing out possible problems with the performance of infusion devices (MDA, 2000 and 2002a) and the following year also published a Device Bulletin devoted to infusion pumps and systems (MDA, 2003). The 2000 document, for example, emphasised problems with the use of devices, such as:

> infusion pumps have been mistaken for each other ... lack of training or lack of familiarity with the set-up and programming of the particular model ... serious problems arise as a result of failure to check the correct flow rates.
>
> (MDA, 2000)

The UK MDA targeted health professionals in a booklet setting out principles for the use and purchasing of medical devices in general (MDA, 2000). By way of introduction, the Agency referred to the growing sophistication of medical devices and to clinical governance as part of the regulatory environment: 'Coupled with modern self-regulation there is emphasis on the accountability of both the individual and the organisation to provide a working environment that supports provision of safe and effective care for patients'. It is significant that in a section called 'People Make Errors', the Agency chose to present infusion pumps as a prime example used to highlight the implications of trends in medical device innovation for health professionals' accountabilities. It is pointed out that 'in addition to the burden of knowledge that a death or serious injury could have been avoided by the correct use of a device', increasingly the coroner refers such fatalities to the police. The users who set up and calibrate infusion pumps, the Agency noted, are usually nurses and midwives. The document goes on to give the following example:

> A report was received from a coroner of user error resulting in a fatality. An infusion rate of 20mm per hour was set instead of 2mm per hour. The practitioner who had set up the pump had not been trained in the use of the pump ... No fault was found with the pump nor was there any data in its memory to indicate a cause of the reported over-infusion. The possibility of user error in setting up the pump has been strongly suggested.
>
> (MDA, 2000)

Bearing in mind the illustrations of what we have called usership science in this chapter, it is clear that this framing of pump performance problems was towards the identification of users' competence. As we have already suggested, and as we demonstrate below, this type of construction of error is being re-shaped by emerging governance in this field.

Regulation has also been developed through direct, independent testing of devices. Between 2003 and 2005, the UK national Device Evaluation Centre for infusion pumps published many studies about the performance of specific models of the device (See, for example Davey, 2003a; Davey, 2003b; Hill, 2003; Bath Institute of Medical Engineering (BIME), 2003; Dunn, 2004a, 2004b; Skryabina, 2004; Davey, 2005). These documents provide a brief description for devices on the UK market of electromechanical features, pointing out novel technical features, advantages and disadvantages, faults during testing, evaluator assessment of ergonomics, a sample-based user assessment of the interface, manufacturer's data, test methods and protocols and manufacturer's comments about the tests. They therefore give extensive coverage to issues of functionality, safe use with patients and effective operation.

The industry producing infusion devices also involves itself in the regulation of their use. For example, Baxter International in a notice of 2005 'alerted customers to several user interface and error code issues with Colleague models that have the potential to disrupt infusions of intravenous therapies'. The company had responded by 'modifying the design of the infusion pump software to reduce the possibility of inadvertently powering off the device when starting an infusion, and to make the pump more fault tolerant'. Other responses to apparent faults may evoke recommendations from the supplying company for users to use the device in a new way or with special attention to certain features. For example, a Device Alert from the MHRA for Baxter Colleague Volumetric pump in 2005–6 notified various problems and Baxter's remedial measures or advice to remove the device from service. The complex, contestable socio-technological issues of attributing responsibility for error is illustrated by the company's responses, such as: 'To avoid an obstruction during IV administration set loading: Ensure that when loading the IV administration set, the tubing is loaded along the entire length of the tubing channel to avoid a misload or incomplete load situation' (MHRA, 2006).

Incident reports show that infusion/transfusion/dialysis devices have a slowly rising trend of reports of adverse incidents in the UK (MHRA, 2006). In addition to this, NPSA-collected data showed an estimated one in ten patients to be involved in such incidents, which 'are often minor and transient', and of which 'research has suggested up to half ... are avoidable'. In 2004 the UK Department of Health policy document on safer medication (DoH, 2004) reported that between 1990 and 2000 in the UK, 6773 adverse incident reports associated with infusion and transfusion devices had been received by the MDA, including 85 fatalities (MDA, 2003). The document states unequivocally that 'user error' was the most common identifiable cause (Department of Health, 2004: 102). As noted above (section in this chapter on regulatory divergence), an investigation of 1495 incidents directly related to infusion pumps revealed that in 53 per cent of cases there was no fault found with the device and that the error rate attributed to users was nearly three times higher with infusion pumps than with other medical devices.

As the data presented above show, the different regulatory and policy agencies have produced somewhat conflicting diagnoses of the sources of infusion pump incidents. In 2004, the NPSA in the UK made this issue a priority and funded an infusion device project. This was a flagship project closely tied into the initial construction of the NPSA's identity and remit. Other stakeholders enrolled included the NHS PASA (NHS PASA, 2005), MHRA, the national device evaluation centre for infusion devices (BIME) and the Royal College of Nursing (RCN). The aims of the project were to assess the proliferation of the technology, identify the scope of infusion pump–related problems, to analyse the problems and to recommend measures for improvement.

In six pilot hospitals/NHS Trusts starting in 2002, the project assessed the diffusion of the technology. There were 121 infusion devices on the market. They found 1065 devices in use, and an average 31 different types of pumps in each hospital. During a one-year period the six pilot sites reported no deaths, but 321 patient safety incidents, which were classified as 96 over-infusion, 21 under-infusion, 12 device failure and 10 tampering episodes – all by patients, and 59 classified as '*use* error' (NPSA, 2004a). The pilot sites introduced schemes to improve aspects of innovation and use of the device including user training, purchasing practices, incident reporting and risk management systems.

Standardising the way the devices are used, stored and maintained, and reducing the range of devices were concluded as the main policies to reduce errors. The agency is also developing an e-learning pro-gramme to give staff better training. From an engineering point of view, lack of standardisation of software, interface and procedures would appear to be soluble by design changes. The NPSA strategy has been to seek standardisation through the buying process instead of by trying to influence design directly. One of the outcomes of the project was a 'purchasing toolkit':

> Changing the design ... and get some kind of standardised interface – that's too ambitious, so we ruled the purchasing. And ... it takes years to get a standard item and then regulation, so some sort of enforced standardisation by purchasing these models is a good way for standardisation and to force the industry to think. If nobody buys upside-down keypads then the manufacturer who makes upside-down keypads will either stop making them or go bust, either way it's (good) for the market.
>
> (interview with NPSA official, 20 March 2006)

Views about the success of the project in the wider healthcare system varied. Our fieldwork in the UK agencies showed that some NPSA regulatory officials believed that the outcome would be poor if the government did not invest in replacing old pumps in the hospitals. It was felt that impact depended also on efforts to change hospital and industry procedures.

Professional guidelines and standards for medication have also been produced during the period in which the patient safety agenda has developed. Standards have been developed, for example, by the RCN

(RCN, 2003). These standards and training courses associated with them are framed in terms of the whole procedure of IV medication, so they cover not only the use of infusion devices but also general competence in IV therapy, theory of drip rate and drug calculations, principles of fluid and electrolyte therapy, risks management and managing risks of IV therapy and infection control.

Patient safety has also been constituted as an issue in EU health policy. A system-based approach to patient safety is espoused (European Health Committee, 2005). This policy, like that underpinning the NPSA, draws on academic literature on industrial and organisational accidents (for example, Vincent et al., 1998). European Health Committe policy (op. cit., 2005) identifies a large number of arenas in which scientific research is required in the general area of patient safety. These include: descriptive, qualitative studies of patient safety incidents in all health care settings; epidemiologic studies to identify risk factors for patient safety incidents; involving patients; patient safety indicators; experimental research on 'human factors' and 'human error'; evaluation of effectiveness of interventions to improve patient safety; FMEA and other tools and methods of education.

The devices industry at European level has also involved itself in infusion pumps policy. For example, medical devices trade association Eucomed has planned a position statement on this family of devices (Eucomed, 2008). The statement addresses areas for action such as establishment of systematic and efficient incident reporting systems at national level within a 'no blame' culture, centralised training for nurses, standardisation, international harmonised standards, adequate maintenance by hospitals of infusion devices and responsible hospital purchasing policies.

There is thus a complex patchwork of different regulatory agencies and stakeholders at different levels engaging in a wide variety of safety assessment, information-gathering, monitoring, policy-formulation and regulatory activity. Among these governance actors, there are diverging framings of policy goals and diverging understandings of the criteria for technology evaluation. However, one clear trend is towards gatekeeping of the point of purchase. We now consider this development in the case of the UK.

Procurement as regulation

There is a movement among the UK policymaking actors, seen also, for example, in the case of artificial hips, to marshal gatekeeping controls at the points of purchase of equipment. There are several manifestations of this trend. The two agencies that are leading this in the UK are the NPSA and the NHS PASA.

The NPSA has developed a toolkit to help NHS trusts review their existing device management systems, as well as assess the potential for significant cost benefits. Their guidance for the policy of an NHS Trust purchasing infusion equipment in the mid-2000s is that there should be, firstly, a review of how purchasing decisions are made; secondly, an evaluation of the necessity for an infusion device before it is purchased; thirdly, reduction in the range of infusion device types in use, and that within each type there should be locally agreed default configurations; and fourthly, the benefits of a centralised equipment library should be investigated.

In 2005 and 2006 the agency had received around 800 reports per month on incidents relating to injectable medicines. Early in 2007, NPSA issued a series of specific medication-related 'safety alerts'. Government ministers discussed possible actions to counter what appeared to be a rising trend. This resulted in a recommendation for NHS PASA to implement and fund pilot sites within the NHS to test 'Purchasing for Safety' benefits in the area of injectable medicines (NHS PASA, 2007). A pilot project in four NHS Trusts began in 2007 with the aim to demonstrate that strategic purchasing can reduce clinical risk associated with the administration of injectable medicines, to learn lessons relating to injectable medicines of benefit to trusts and collaborative procurement hubs[4] and to develop a model for wider government policy through procurement. The objectives of the scheme include reduction of risk via design and labelling of products; standardisation of technology, supporting training and protocols; reduction of medicines requiring complex calculation and increased use of ICT-based double checking systems such as bar-coding and electronic dose limiting software.

Companies such as Baxter International are participating in this project: 'Baxter supports the NHS in advancing patient safety by continuously innovating treatments and the delivery of care for people with critical conditions' (Baxterhealthcare, 2006). The company claims it has invested significant funds to provide clinical, cost-effectiveness data and evidence in areas such as medical device standardisation and risk reduction in the preparation of IV therapy.

As noted in Chapter 3 of this book, a key move in reconfiguring the institutional regime of device regulation has been to move the scientific device evaluation service out of the MHRA, the authority responsible for implementing the EU device regulations, and into the national purchasing agency NHS PASA. The move is doubly significant because, first, it is part of the NHS rather than an agency of the government Department of Health, and, second, its jurisdiction is for purchasing policy. The boundary between the national agency of the EU regulatory system and the national purchasing agency is a site of friction and contested construction of the market-worthiness of device technologies, as we pointed out above in discussing the 'evaluation gap':

> devices assessed by the Device Evaluation Service are already CE marked, and therefore deemed fit for purpose. However, the essential requirements for CE marking do not currently address usability in significant detail.
>
> (Dunn et al., 2006)

The relocation of national-level device evaluation services thus highlights the issue of the type of evidence that might be produced in the name of 'evidence-based purchasing'. The study by Dunn referred to above was conducted under the auspices of the national Device Evaluation Service, and it aimed to apply and improve a usability assessment tool for application to infusion devices already available on the market. The aim was to provide a tool to improve hospital or regional purchasers' resources for assessing and selecting equipment. The CEP advises that a range of people should be involved in purchasing for an NHS Trust, including clinicians and equipment managers. If done at regional level it advises that the NHS Procurement Hubs may coordinate this. Existing evaluation reports from PASA may help in assessing the tenders produced by potential suppliers (for example, CEP, 2007).

The role of patient safety in the device purchasing process, with infusion pumps taken as the focus, has also been the subject of analysis in the advanced healthcare systems of other countries. A 'human factors' interview-based study has been reported in New York hospital purchasing divisions (Johnson et al., 2005). The study identified similar dimensions of the safety issues at the point of purchasing as the UK NPSA analysis. Interestingly, the authors suggested that FDA approval is interpreted by many purchasing decision makers as ensuring safety of devices – a similar analysis to that implied by Dunn et al.'s statement quoted above about CE-marking.

Hospital pharmacists also play a part in purchasing policy and decisions. The risk assessment undertaken by a hospital pharmacy procurement group is likely increasingly to include safety criteria. These criteria can embrace concerns about the usability of medicines, for example through labelling and packaging. Making safety one of the criteria for awarding contracts to suppliers has reportedly met with a mixed response from the pharmaceutical industry, with resistance coming from big pharmaceutical companies. However, the NPSA, the MHRA and the NHS PASA have all been supportive of the policy, according to an account of debate among the Procurement and Distribution Interest Group of the Guild of Healthcare Pharmacists in the UK (Jones, 2003). The MHRA has moved to recommend that hospital trusts should establish multidisciplinary infusion systems committees who should advise on standardisation of infusion equipment, procurement, as well as methods of use, training and maintenance. Such groups should include representatives from pharmacy, medical engineering, supplies and medical and nursing representatives from a range of clinical specialities (Department of Health, 2004).

Thus it is clear that in the UK the possible governance leverage that might be generated by influencing the purchasing and procurement process is the object of substantial development, experimentation and evaluation, and it appears that this tactic together with the system-level focus of the purposefully designed NPSA have become key parts of a governance arena in which there are known gaps in the coverage of the statutory regulatory and evaluatory regimes. Thus the NHS has found a way to address problems with the safety and quality of electromedical equipment produced under the European medical devices regulation without directly confronting the infusion pump industry. By aiming to standardise through purchasing, the NHS tries to keep its patients protected without colliding with MHRA and the powerful CE-marking model.

Dynamics of infusion pump innovation and governance

The evaluation of infusion pump innovation into healthcare has been the subject of a pattern of governance attentions and inattentions. A co-constitution of infusion pump usership and a governance discourse of performance framed in terms of patient safety have been illustrated in this chapter. The governance pattern is complex in ways specific to this type of technology, with its mixture of electrical, mechanical and software features, its interfaces with human users and with digital communication and information systems and its association with life-supporting specialised medication.

The nursing profession especially has found itself in the line of fire when it comes to combining professional accountabilities with framings of user error. A measure of self-regulation through training and sub-specialisation is evident here, the latter appearing to be more developed in the US than the UK, with, for example, a specialist *Journal of Infusion Nursing* now being published. Nursing perspectives and their professional association were prominent in defining the agenda of the NPSA in the UK, with its emphasis on blame-free culture, development of risk management techniques and system-level analysis. The various regulatory actors have converged to some extent in identifying procurement as a gatekeeping point at which multidisciplinary professional groups may exert a regulatory influence over the diversification of technologies in the healthcare workplace.

It is clear that while various stakeholders produce a great deal of scientific and regulatory data classified in different ways, their interpretations of infusion pump technology and practice should be understood as discursive constructions designed to achieve a variety of aims such as better control, fulfilment of legally defined roles, better management, reduction of risk, quicker innovation into the healthcare system, standardisation and so on. Thus we can point to the apparent contradiction between the high profile given to the notion of 'user error', implying deficiencies in learning and competence, which has been joined latterly by the notion of 'system failure' and the notion of 'usability' in post-market device evaluation, which implies a mixture of governance through technology design and user competence. The recent software-dependent technological innovations embodied in smart pumps appear to address user error and usability. Beyond, but closely linked to these framings of evaluations of the usership of infusion pump technology, is the growing regulatory attention to the complexity of the technological working environment, particularly gatekeeping of its entry-points:

The general requirements for (EU) medical device directives is to minimise as far as possible the risk of injury to staff and patients. And then use inherently safe design. And I would say the way we have chosen to interpret things has been rather minimal. ... On a personal level I would say it's [my relation with MHRA] poor. ... Because my message is not one ... they particularly want to hear. Because I am saying to them I believe X device is actually unsafe and this is a device that they have tested and said that's suitable. So I'm saying from a design perspective it's so cumbersome, so complex and difficult for the user to use that I don't feel it complies with the medical devices directives in the way that I interpret them. And that's not a message that they really see as part of our remit.

(NPSA official, 20/03/2006)

This statement highlights issues of ambiguity in the perceptions of juris-dictions among the relevant regulatory actors. The NPSA official is drawing on an institutionally shaped construction of usership that indicates the significance of the UK government's reconfiguration of 'technical' device evaluation, represented by the moving of the national Device Evaluation centres from the arena of devices regulation (MHRA) to the arena of purchasing and procurement (NHS PASA). As with other medical devices, the statutory European regulatory system relies more on post-marketing vigilance (reporting and collation of incident data on alleged failures) than it does on market approval under the devolved and partly self-certifying system. If an infusion pump 'delivers the wrong dose because of an incompatibility between the pump and the infusion set used (and) if the combination of pump and set used was in accordance with the instructions for use' the manufacturer should report the failure to the authority (EC DG Enterprise & Industry, 2007).

Thus there are clashing perspectives on safety criteria at the ill-defined boundaries between the two key agencies involved in assessing, moni-toring and attempting to shape the process of healthcare innovation. It is clear that in the UK the 'patient safety' agency's construction of the concept of technological safety proceeds from different normative assumptions about, especially, the usability dimension of device safety. Both agencies have made recommendations about training in the use of pumps, and the NPSA has focused more upon understandings of error grounded in 'systems' and organisational approaches to analysing the sources of error. A more recent development is that of 'usability stan-dards', and it seems clear that the there will be continued jurisdictional friction around attempts at shaping infusion pump usership.

It is notable, comparing this case study to the others in this book, that a scientific evaluation of 'effectiveness' and cost-effectiveness via the HTA regime is conspicuously absent. The UK-based NICE is reviewing implantable insulin infusion therapy and there has been HTA-mode assessment of this technology. The absence of appraisal of external, bedside infusion pump technology is partly to be explained by the char-acteristics of the material technology itself. As a functional device, the infusion pump is a vehicle for delivering medical material of one sort or another to the human body, and so it is not a therapeutic intervention in itself. Also, the technology is deployed in a very wide range of medical conditions and healthcare settings, and it is likely that it would only be assessed, if at all, as part of a restricted field of clinical applica-tion. Also, of course, the basic technology is already well embedded into healthcare practice. The evaluation of the cost-effectiveness of pilot introductions of smart pumps, however, is a potential candidate for controlled trial or other HTA evaluation.

Issues of industry-supported proliferation and diversification of technologies, at the level of the healthcare delivery institution and regional organisation, and issues of usership and usability at the level of professional practice, dominate the pathways of innovation and governance of infusion pump technology. In this case study we have analysed the key institutional and discursive vectors along which these innovation/governance issues are being shaped. We now turn to a brief consideration of this case study in terms of the theoretical technology-in-healthcare-in-society concerns of this book.

Infusion pump technology and society

The infusion pump innovation pathway provides a number of particular features for an analysis of society/technology relations, medicalisation, usership, evidentiality and state intervention. Infusion pumps are highly 'social' in use. The sociality of the technology lies in the complex nexus of medico-social and medico-organisational relationships in which a functionally complex device is deployed, and in which its usership by health professionals is constructed.

Medicalisation takes several forms in the case of this technology. It has been shown that concepts of pain and the disciplinary regimes of healthcare have changed over the last decades partly through technological developments of which infusion pumps are one example (Winslow et al., 2003). Public concern about the technology surfaces when health and life-threatening incidents occur. Through the massive regulatory construction of this as an issue and the response to it, the device has become associated with what has been called the rise of a 'safety culture' in western society. In the UK, the invention of a dedicated patient safety agency is a key indicator of this. Medicalisation reshapes healthcare expertise and organisation, and the part played by the biomedical devices industry here is of obvious significance. The innovative smart pumps and networking technologies promoted by industry, paradoxically, could increase standardisation and reduce the number of different device types, and different manufacturers' presence, in a healthcare setting. This may not be a pathway that healthcare policymakers would wish to encourage because it would represent an increase in the coupling of skills and knowledge to particular proprietary technologies. Such an analysis gives some specification to aspects of the biomedicalisation thesis (Clarke et al., 2003) and the corporatisation thesis of medicalisation (Conrad, 2005).

Infusion pump–related discourse shows a *technologically* driven construction of population, patient and societal risk. It is evident that the concept of safety itself is more likely to be evoked with some technologies than others. Technological safety risk, as with infusion devices, is construed through particular alignments between material technology, the mediating institutions of sciences and the state and social actors. Indeed, the voice of citizen-patients has been largely absent from this account of infusion technology, which suggests that the regulatory-scientific actors described here act *in loco civis*, the state attempting to shape technological innovation on behalf of citizens. This can be seen as one form of custodianship.

This account of infusion pumps revolves around usership and technological complexity: users' skills, knowledge and technical expertise; governance: the management of risks associated with use of the devices; the social and organisational contexts of use of the device; science: the detailed study and attempted explanation of the safety and dangers of its use; technological innovation: the building-in for users of aids to expertise, communications and safety. In terms of social shaping, technological scripting of users and the creative domestication of technology, we can see that infusion pump innovation has aspects that accord with each of these perspectives. Infusion pump technology embeds not only 'users' in the sense of aggregates of people who operate the device, but also – in the technology of networked smart infusion pumps – 'society' in the sense of models of interrelationships between different individuals and different organised working groups. Clinical engineers who customise pumps to block out the smart drug library–based features actively 'domesticate' the technology; nurse-users in a usability study act as design participants – users who are both configured by technology and have the capacity to configure at least some aspects of it. With its increasing incorporation of software features and electronic connectivity, infusion pumps exhibit signs of a growing distributedness of the patient body characteristic of broad trends within healthcare towards 'informaticisation' and e-health (Webster, 2002, 2007: 10–13).

In the UK the NPSA has conceived a more social or sociological and organisational analysis of interactions between infusion pumps and healthcare systems and health professionals than would be allowed in the discourse of a regulatory agency working in the EU device regime. Indeed, the architects of the patient safety agendas have explicitly seen themselves as constructing the scaffolding (information systems, reporting procedures, risk managers for a learning organisation) – of an 'organisation with a memory'. The conceptualisation of systems underlying errors is indeed consistent with well known organisational and sociological analysis that has identified 'normal accidents' as a feature of complex techno-organisational systems (Perrow, 1999; Collins and Pinch, 1998). It is epitomised here by the distinction between *user* error and *use* error. Thus a 'social learning' model of infusion pump development and diffusion is highly appropriate to *this* technology (Stewart and Williams, 2005).

In this governance arena we see a construction of 'users' proceeding from a formulation of the healthcare system and its staff as a learning organisation rather than as an aggregate of operators of technology, to an extent which suggests that the concept of the 'user', whether passive or active, individual or collectively organised, may not be appropriate at all. When we attempt to understand how usership is inscribed into and around technological artefacts, therefore, as we do in Science and Technology Studies, we would perhaps better conceptualise this strand of the conundrum of technology and society more in terms of the configuring of *social actors* rather than merely 'users', no matter how active and inventive we might be *as* users.

7
Coagulometers: Healthcare Governance at Home

Introduction

Coagulometers are used for measuring and monitoring the viscosity of blood. Some models are designed to be operated by laboratory staff or health professionals, while some recent models are small and portable and can be operated by the end-users – patients themselves. Coagulometer technology in different forms can thus be used in pathology laboratories, in primary care settings or by patients either at home or while travelling. The devices, commercially available, produce information that can be used with patients undergoing drug therapy for a variety of heart and circulatory conditions that might produce potentially dangerous blood clotting. The device is used, therefore, in the context of a number of life-threatening medical conditions. The development of portable versions of the device is relatively recent, and thus it appears in a context in which other technologies and particular specialised forms of health professional expertise and organisation are already institutionalised.

The case of coagulometers is particularly interesting in a comparative analysis of medical devices because, unlike the other cases discussed in this book, there is a strong, organised patient advocacy movement to promote the direct use of this device by patients, at home or mobile. Unlike many health technologies, the end-users are active patients who engage with operation and interpretation of the device. Allied to patient advocacy, coagulometers can be seen also as part of a growing range of 'self-care' techniques and technologies that to some extent may substitute for and enable decentralised healthcare services, and in principle may empower service users. This trend is strongly aligned with international policy movements that seek to support empowerment of patients and decentralisation of healthcare services delivery. 'Do-It-Yourself' anticoagulation monitoring raises important questions of expertise, responsibility for risk, accountabilities and the re-structuring of health-care delivery and governance.

The main focus of the chapter is the coagulometer device as used by people who monitor their own anticoagulation therapy, and, in some cases, manage their own medication regime. Technical evaluations and the clinical evidence of healthcare science are summarised and the impetus behind the production of this evidence is discussed. The development of coagulometer technology is outlined, including the role of industry. Some international variation in the healthcare policy on these devices is noted. The chapter discusses modes of communication between patients and health professionals in the UK and some evidence of users' experience of the technology. It analyses the ways in which the clinical evidence about effectiveness is produced and deployed by clinical, patient-user and industry stakeholders, and it shows resistances in the UK healthcare system to widespread adoption. As with previous chapters, the nature of the technology is analysed for its implications for governance and socio-medical diffusion.

Epidemiology and the marketplace

Hundreds of thousands of people worldwide take drugs for blood thinning in order to treat or prevent heart and circulatory conditions. The actual number is probably in the order of seven million. It is estimated that some 950,000 people currently use long-term oral anti-coagulation therapy (OAT) in the UK. Chronic medical conditions for which blood-thinning drugs (mainly warfarin in the UK) may be administered include heart disease, deep vein thrombosis (DVT), stroke and patients with artificial heart valves following cardiac surgery. It is believed that the number using OAT could be much larger if a higher percentage of people suffering atrial fibrillation (AF – irregular contractions of the heart muscles), who are at risk of suffering a stroke, were to use medication.

Coagulation must be controlled to prevent haemorrhaging or heart failure. Blood clotting in the brain could cause a stroke; in the heart it could cause a heart attack; in the leg, gangrene; in the lung, pulmonary embolism Anticoagulants can be used by people at risk of developing clots, such as those with certain inherited disorders or after injury or surgery. The ageing population and high incidence of heart and circulatory conditions indicate that demand for health service resources for monitoring and treatment will continue to rise. Issues of access to the new technologies and service models include variations according to ethnicity: Indian/Asian and African–origin people require higher warfarin dosage than whites, with implications for device usage, software design and training.

Available evidence supports long-term treatment with vitamin K antagonists (counteracting drugs) such as warfarin. Warfarin is the most widely used oral anticoagulant and can be administered in tablet form. In the UK it is commonly available under the brand name Marevan (marketed by Goldshield, a British-based pharmaceutical and healthcare products company[1], and it is also on the market as a generic drug. In other countries other brand names are found, for example Coumadin is common in the USA, Apo-Warfarin among others in Canada and Jantoven, Panwarfin, Waran and Sofarin are also to be found[2]. The appropriate dose must be individualised because patients react differently to warfarin, and the same patient may react differently over time. If the dose is too low, a patient may be inadequately protected against developing a blood clot. If the dose is too high, the risk of bleeding or haemorrhaging is increased. This creates a need for monitoring the degree of anticoagulation in patients on long-term OAT. Monitoring can be achieved through the use of coagulometer technologies.

Development of anticoagulation monitoring and the coagulometer

Anticoagulation monitoring

In order to understand the working of anticoagulation monitoring devices, and thus the knowledge and expertise that the technology's users might require, it is necessary to understand how blood viscosity is measured. A method for producing a standardised measurement of coagulation internationally was introduced in the early 1980s, called the International Normalized Ratio, referred to as INR. It has had the endorsement of the WHO since 1983. The INR is the ratio of the patient's prothrombin time (PT) compared to the mean prothrombin time for a group of normal individuals. Prothrombin time is defined as the time it takes blood plasma to clot after addition of tissue factor (a protein important to thrombin formation). Prothrombin time is prolonged in the case of deficiencies of vitamin K, and can alter in relation to diet, stress and other lifestyle factors. The INR is the ratio of a patient's prothrombin time to a normal sample, raised to the power of the 'ISI' mean population value (Figure 7.1). Each manufacturer gives an

$$INR = \left(\frac{PT_{test}}{PT_{normal}} \right)^{ISI}$$

Figure 7.1 Definition of INR (International Normalized Ratio) measure of anticoagulation status

ISI (International Sensitivity Index) for any tissue factor they produce. The ISI value indicates how any given batch of tissue factor compares to an internationally standardised sample.

The result of the INR algorithm applied to any single test result is a number, and it is this which is the focus of the clinical and patient user's attention in understanding their coagulation level and the possible need for an adjustment of the dose of warfarin. For patients with AF, an INR of 2.0–3.0 may be appropriate and for those with an artificial heart valve, 2.5–3.5. An INR generally less than 2.0 is associated with an increased risk of thromboembolism due to clotting, while an INR of more than 4.5 is associated with increase in the risk of major bleeding.

A typical haematology clinic regime for adjustment of warfarin therapy depending upon INR readings is as shown in Table 7.1.

Table 7.1 Typical haematology recommendations for warfarin therapy

INR	Warfarin adjustment
1.0 − 1.5	50% increase
1.5 − 2.0	30% increase
2.0 − 3.0	*No change*
3.0 − 3.5	15% reduction
3.5 − 4.0	20% reduction
4.0 − 6.0	25% reduction
6.0 − 8.0	Stop for 2 days and 33% reduction

Assuming a target INR of 2.0 to 3.0.

The 'therapeutic range' in which safety is indicated is thus very narrow, making the performance and use of any monitoring technology critical.

Coagulometer technology

'Near-patient testing' or 'point-of-care' versions of anticoagulation monitoring technology have been developed for use in outreach services or services based in primary care service settings. An increasing range of new generation machines and reagents using computerised decision-support software is gaining clinical acceptance. I do not discuss near-patient technologies in detail here, preferring to concentrate on what I take to be the technological development with more radical implications, namely the self-monitoring device and the possibility of patients managing their own drug regime.

Small hand-held coagulometers are made possible by advances in miniaturisation, solid phase chemistry and software. INR self-monitoring began in the mid-1980s, in Germany, with a monitor that required about half an hour to operate. German company, Boehringer Mannheim (now Roche Diagnostics) launched the first self-monitoring device 'CoaguChek' in 1994. This technology continues to be developed, and monitoring time has been reduced to a few minutes.

Manufacturers claim that the technology has fail-safe features including automatic control of internal system functions, and results are displayed only after several quality control steps. Also required to perform the monitoring are test strips containing a reagent, lancets for obtaining fingertip blood and a quality control liquid solution. Of the several types of coagulometer commercially available, there are several different modes of operation, not detailed here. All systems produce the INR level as a readout on a display screen in the device. Technological developments for point-of-care devices include incorporation of dosing software and audit trail systems for linking patients' data items into patient databases in healthcare provider IT systems. A 'home-made' anti-coagulation monitor has been reported (in Austria – Finsterer, et al., 2000), initially with good results, followed by negative later assessment.

Related to the technology of the coagulometer itself is the technology of communicating between coagulometer user and health professionals in the healthcare system. Advances in database and communications technology are promoting a widespread increase in opportunities for near-patient diagnosis, testing and self-management. The Royal College of General Practitioners recently recommended use of computerised decision-support systems in primary care–based anticoagulation services, and use of computer-assisted dose control in primary care is increasing. There is a growing concern about a proliferation of methods of communicating between primary care and hospital.

Coagulation self-monitoring may be regarded from a clinical-healthcare system perspective as a 'distance technology' (Balas and Iakovidis 1999). It is thus part of the family of technologies of telemedicine or telehealth. Such systems assume that the health professional and the patient are in different locations, and possibly at different points in time, at the time of the medical episode. The introduction of telemedicine technologies into healthcare systems has been far less extensive than many early commentators predicted (May et al., 2003a). The coagulometer as a distance technology does not require connectivity between, for example, a visual display device and a camera at a remote location. Self-monitoring patients will typically be required by medical professionals to remain connected *to some extent* to regimes of care in a clinic-based system. This revolves around the recording and communication of INR readings to the health professional, whether in primary care or hospital-based clinic. Traditionally, the readings are recorded in a booklet given to the patient.

An EU-supported telemedicine approach has been piloted and evaluated in the UK (Gardiner et al., 2006), reportedly showing acceptable 'user-friendliness' and a need for technical testing *in situ*. In general, however, there is a paucity of research on the implications of communication media and information flows with coagulometers, regardless of the care setting. Further proliferation of communication media is likely, some of which will seek empowerment of patients to communicate their INR data to the clinic, e.g., by mobile phone text messaging as already evaluated in the case of blood glucose monitoring for people with diabetes (Vahatalo et al., 2004). The viability of linkage of self-monitoring and self-managing data to patients' electronically stored other medical records is an obvious issue to be explored.

The industry

Medical device companies herald a movement to increase the use of self-testing technologies (Anon, 2004). A small number of medical diagnostic equipment manufacturers are currently in the self-testing anticoagulation field. The market has been forecast to rise from €140m in 2003 to €350m in 2009 (Anon., op. cit.).

The most common proprietary coagulometer in the UK and other advanced healthcare systems is the 'Coaguchek', produced in a succession of models by Roche Diagnostics. It can store 60 INR readings at once. One advertisement claimed: 'Home warfarin testing at your fingertips'. Roche Diagnostics has its headquarters in (Mannheim) Germany. As noted, the device was originally developed by Boehringer Mannheim GmbH, a German company that Roche took over in 1998[3]. Roche is a Swiss company and globally it is the largest company in the diagnostics healthcare market, with the broadest product range. Roche claims over 10,000 users of the coagulometer in the UK in 2007, and 250,000 worldwide. The company involves itself in clinical centres: 'Collaborates with UK national centre for anticoagulation training' and provides support services for users, via the 'Coaguchek Care Line'. The company also has some involvement with patient organisations in the field.

A small number of other devices exist. The Roche market-leading product has been joined since 2003 by a device produced in the USA called INRatio™, produced by the company HemoSense, which manufactures only this device. It is CE-marked and so can be marketed in the EU. As noted in the section below on regulation, this device, like the Roche devices, has been formally evaluated in the UK through the government-mandated Device Evaluation Centre system. There are thus early signs of expansion of commercial producers of this technology.

Policy and governance

Coagulometer technology is part of a developing policy field. Most obviously, the technology is supportive of broader societal movements to promote individual autonomy, empowerment, self-efficacy, non-dependence, personal expertise and the like. On the other hand, because the technology is used in the context of high-risk medical conditions, the growing movement among governments and healthcare policymakers to improve healthcare safety practices and cultures is a counteracting trend. Allied to these trends, the growth of regulatory evidentiality is also conspicuous in the innovation of INR self-monitoring into advanced industrial healthcare systems.

Self-care and the expert patient

Self-care and 'expert patient' initiatives are major policy initiatives in the NHS in the UK. The UK Government convened an Expert Patients Task Force in 1999 and the resulting report recommended action over a 6- year period to introduce lay-led self-management training programmes (Department of Health, 2001a). From 2002 to 2004 all primary care trusts in England were to pilot self-management activity and from 2004 to 2007 the programme was included in the mainstream of healthcare provision in the NHS. Although there is debate about the value of these programmes (Kennedy et al., 2003), the discourse of self-care is thus becoming widely embedded in healthcare system strategy. Anticoagulation self-monitoring is not included in the government-supported expert patient programmes.

Coagulometer policy

Some countries such as Germany have actively introduced home monitoring technologies, including the full cost of reimbursement, but other countries such as the UK and Spain have been less enthusiastic. In UK debates the example of Germany is very frequently referred to. In Europe, Denmark, the Netherlands and Austria also have full reimbursement cover. The reason why Germany has introduced the technology so widely is partly that legal framework conditions have enabled health insurance companies to provide patients with coagulometers free of charge. Doctors in that country appear to have welcomed INR self-management due to a perceived significantly improved compliance with treatment regimes (Schaeffer, 2007). The US, perhaps surprisingly, has been a relatively cautious innovator. US reimbursement is limited to only patients with mechanical heart valves. The medical professions are reported to have concerns about liability for untoward events, about instrument accuracy and a low level of awareness that such therapy is available (Ansell, 2007).

The handheld coagulometer devices are not supplied currently via the UK NHS. Patient advocacy groups such as the British Cardiac Patients Association (BCPA) and Anticoagulation Europe (ACE) are prominent in promoting self-management, linking with manufacturers and clinician-champions, raising funds for coagulometers, being represented on Department of Health policy groups and negotiating on policy issues, such as the NHS prescription status for testing strips.

Policy in the UK in this field is piecemeal and local practices vary widely. A small number of hospital-based clinical centres are known to support local initiatives, but these are uncoordinated. A number of resistances to self-monitoring can be identified, and areas that require further evaluation. These include patient and clinical acceptability, selection criteria for patients, NHS commitment to and targeting of self-testing devices and the generalisability of the modest evidence base.

Regulation and regulatory science

Coagulometers (manufacturers) are regulated within the EU as diagnostic medical devices under the In Vitro Diagnostic Device Directive, which was transposed into UK law in 2000. They must, therefore, have been certified though the Notified Bodies system (see Chapter 3, on medical device regulation). The Directive requires that devices for self-testing must take into account the likely level of skill of the intended user and the influence on the test result that could come from variation in technique and environment. Information and instructions for use should be easily understood and applied, and should state that decisions about medical treatment should not be taken without consultation with a medical practitioner. As with other types of device, adverse incidents and potential problems should be reported to the competent authority, in the UK the MHRA. Guidance may be produced, or in serious instances, a 'medical device alert' to prevent the multiplication of problems.

For example, in the UK community pharmacists were recently involved in managing the consequences of a defect in the foil packaging of a batch of coagulometer test strips that could have led to dangerously misleading INR readings (MHRA, 2005).

The MHRA has a growing concern with self-testing technology, including 'over-the-counter' kits. Thus they have produced a Device Bulletin that covers both 'near-patient' testing and self-testing (MHRA, 2002). The aim is to provide guidance on the use of the devices as part of statutory healthcare provision. The Bulletin dealt with issues including the need for training and monitoring of staff, importance of identifying a clinical need before introducing any new service, the need to include 'clinical governance' measures and a need for local hospital pathology laboratory involvement (MHRA, op. cit.).

In the UK the different devices were evaluated by the then MDA as the regulatory authority. Three machines tested were reported to show similar results (CoaguChek/CoaguChek Plus (Roche Diagnostics), TAS/Rapid Point Coag (Bayer Diagnostic) and Protime (International Technidyne Corporation)). All three machines showed comparable INRs across the therapeutic range (Fitzmaurice and Machin, 2001). Accuracy and reproducibility of results and long-term use by patients was good (Bhavnani and Shiach, 2002). The evolving forms of the Coaguchek have been studied extensively by the UK regulatory agencies. The MHRA published a report from the specialist Device Evaluation Centres (DECs) on a randomised control trial comparing patient self-management with a model in which patients self-monitored, but reported results to a central clinic (Gardiner et al., 2005). The report concluded that the self-management mode was, 'in the majority of suitably trained patients', comparable to self-monitoring patients supported by a specialised centre.

In the UK coagulometers have also been given some priority by the central healthcare products procurement policy agency, the NHS PASA. PASA believes this type of device to be of sufficient importance to have developed a general protocol for their evaluation. Their CEP has evaluated several models, producing reports targeted at the full range of healthcare users and managers. In the case of INRatio, for example, PASA's report on technical functionality concluded that operation was quite simple and no mechanical failures occurred in testing (Longair et al., 2005). When tested against reference standards values, INRs showed 'small but statistically significant differences' of no clinical significance (op. cit., p. 23). In spite of some technical reservations, the report gives the device its seal of approval for safety and usability, for NHS adoption.

Many different professional associations or groups have produced guidance on self-testing practice over the last few years. These include specific international associations, as well as general haematology organisations, such as the British Society of Haematology Task Force for Haemostasis and Thrombosis. This group published revised guidance on oral anticoagulation in 1990, which was criticised by some haematologists as giving too much responsibility to consultant haematologists when GPs could undertake much of the work. The US-based International Self-Monitoring Association for Oral Anticoagulation (ISMAA), a proponent of self-monitoring, produced guidance based on critical review of literature, concluding that it offers: 'a higher degree of medical safety, increased patient education, improved response to changes in lifestyle, increased independence for the patient and improved quality of life' (Ansell et al., 2005). Interestingly, on the contentious point of frequency of testing, this group concluded that: 'lower (than weekly) frequency of testing can be justified', citing 'many studies' (two are referenced) showing more INR results within individuals' therapeutic ranges, correlated with more frequent testing (Ansell, op. cit.). ISMAA has links with commercial medical device/coagulometer companies via educational grants (Ansell, op. cit.), and it is possible that interest bias is operating in this interpretation of the evidence.

There is, therefore, a variety of legislative and less formal regulation affecting coagulometer innovation. In the UK, it is clear that assessment of safety requires consideration also of aspects of the therapeutic milieu in which the device is used. As we will see in the section below on users, this can be a matter of contention for healthcare policy and a matter of negotiation for individual users. In the UK principles of information-sharing and reconfiguration of regulatory agencies have given rise to concern about safety evaluation of coagulometers and their use. For example, the UK's DECs do not have access to the assessment documentation produced by a Notified Body under the auspices of the EU medical device regulatory regime for pre-marketing approval decisions. This may be seen as problematic where self-certification is used, as with all Point-of-Care Testing (POCT) coagulometers (Gardiner, personal communication, 2007). For example, the technical Device Evaluation Service (DES) may find 'serious' calibration problems only after being placed on the market (Gardiner, personal communication 2007). Also, it may be that the institutional re-location of the Device Evaluation Service from regulatory agency MHRA to procurement agency PASA (on the recommendation of the HITF in 2004; see also Chapter 1) may have problematic effects. Thus there is, in these conflicts over the extent and nature of device assessments and their connection with regulatory and purchasing institutions, a complicated set of forces constituting the processes of innovation and evaluation. The institutions and groups involved in these tensions are among the expertise-claiming actors who produce evidence for policy decisions. I now turn to a closer examination of the *clinical* evidence produced about the acceptability of self-monitoring coagulometer devices – the regulatory science of anticoagulation self-monitoring.

Coagulometers are the subject of growing evaluation by regulatory agencies, clinical researchers and professional associations. Limited evidence in the form of narrative accounts of individual patients is also being published by advocacy organisations and proponents of the patient safety agenda. In the UK, the NPSA has investigated hospital-based anticoagulation monitoring but not self-monitoring. Service-oriented evaluation includes assessment of clinical effectiveness and to a lesser extent cost-effectiveness. There is a conspicuous lack of qualitative research investigating phenomenological aspects of patients' experience with these devices and associated reconfiguring of services.

The number of clinical studies of near-patient testing and self-monitoring in this field has been increasing internationally during the last 20 years, although the total number of clinical studies of self-monitoring *per se* is not large: a search of *Embase* using the subject heading/keywords 'self-monitoring' combined with 'anticoagulation' finds hardly any studies published before 1994 (i.e. when the first home-based monitor was introduced), then four between 1995–8, 16 between 1999–2002 and 30 between 2003–6 inclusive (this pattern was confirmed in *Google Scholar*).

Many studies internationally suggest that PSM has equivalent or better control of INR levels. The first RCT of self-management was conducted in 1996, with patients with mechanical heart valves, in one of the main cardiology centres in Europe developing self-management, Ruhr University of Bochum, Bad Oeynhausen, Germany. A number of recent systematic reviews using secondary analysis, including three conducted under the auspices of national or international HTA institutions have recently appeared or are about to. At least two of these include an economic analysis.

One systematic review and meta-analysis conducted under the auspices of the high-status Cochrane Collaboration and published in *The Lancet* consolidates the view that patient self-testing is at least as effective clinically as standard methods (Heneghan et al., 2006). It identified 14 randomised trials of self-monitoring, of which the largest were conducted in Spain, Germany and the USA. The longest period of measurement of outcomes was two years. Meta-analysis of eligible studies showed a reduction in mortality rates, thromboembolisms and major (but not minor) haemorrhage. Heneghan et al., note three previous systematic reviews of self-management alone published from researchers in Norway and Germany (2004) and Spain (2005). These were also supportive.

A UK national HTA programme project aims to assess the evidence for the effectiveness of self-monitoring and self-managing models, together with cost modelling. The study focuses upon the following outcome measures: 'Effectiveness of testing devices; anticoagulation control; adverse events such as bleeding; patient acceptability and satisfaction and compliance; costs to patients and NHS and cost-effectiveness. Also an assessment will be made of appropriate models of care for large populations and specific patient groups and how patients should be identified and trained to self-manage or self-test' (WMHTAC 2007). The HTA study, unlike some such assessments, does not have the status of a 'NICE TAR' – a technology assessment report produced for the regulatory agency NICE. Thus its implications for NICE's recommendations on the technology within the UK healthcare system are not clear. At the same time, the point-of-care device evaluation centre in the UK has been (in 2007) working to produce an individual patient meta-analysis of self-monitoring which will collate data from 20 published trials of self-monitoring.

International studies have also produced supportive findings (for example, Brown et al., 2007, in Canada). One notable finding, indicating some question marks about the user-friendliness of self-monitoring was that (in 6 studies) 12 per cent to 19 per cent of patients abandoned the point-of-care approach during the study. An economic analysis concluded that the point-of-care device was cost-effective from the perspective of society as a whole, but not so from the healthcare provider perspective (a conclusion more negative than some other cost analyses) (Brown et al., op. cit.).

David Fitzmaurice, a primary care specialist and the leading clinical investigator of self-monitoring in the UK, has also undertaken a critical review of published studies of self-monitoring (Fitzmaurice, 2006). Because of the relative lack of research in this area, observational data (that is, studies without control groups) were included as well as controlled trials. He noted that the early studies examined the feasibility of allowing patients receiving oral anticoagulation to undertake self-management and that these were predominantly undertaken in North America.

Controlled trials associated with leading investigators in the UK show that uptake of self-monitoring is higher among younger and more educated patients (and 76 per cent of an unselected group declined self-management – Murray et al, 2004). Fitzmaurice reported the first sizeable trial of self-*management*: 'SMART was the first large-scale UK study to investigate patient self-management of oral anticoagulation. It was primary care based with patients randomised to receive either PSM or standard care only after eligibility for PSM was determined. The principal findings were that around 25 per cent of patients were willing and able to perform PSM, therapeutic control and adverse events were similar to routine care whilst the costs from the NHS perspective were around £350 compared to around £100 for routine care' (Fitzmaurice et al., 2004).

One of the most cited studies in this field internationally is the Germany-based so-called ESCAT study: the 'Early Self Controlled Anticoagulation Trial' (ESCAT I) (Koertke and Koerfer, 2001). This, according to the clinical researchers involved, showed that anticoagulation self-management after mechanical heart valve replacement decreased complication rates by maintaining INR levels closer to the target range than 'home doctor' management.

Proponents of self-management in Germany have undertaken much of the evaluation of training in this field. For example, Sawicki and colleagues in a widely cited evaluation reported a structured programme for patients in 1999, concluding that:

An anticoagulation education program that includes self-management of anticoagulation therapy results in improved accuracy of anticoagulation control and in treatment-related quality-of-life measures.

(Sawicki, 1999)

Sawicki in a 2001 letter to the *British Medical Journal* disputed the modesty of evidence that Fitzmaurice found in trials (Sawicki, 2001), arguing that: 'there is a homogenous evidence from several prospective randomised clinical trials in different countries and settings that after participation in an appropriate teaching and treatment programme, self-management of oral anticoagulation is effective'.

A very wide-ranging and thorough review and policy analysis by the Italian Federation of Anticoagulation Clinics concluded that self-management is possible for some patients, but emphasised that this must be regulated by being based on the existing organisation and skills of its clinics (Fengo et al., 2003). In emphasising specialised quality control, the Italian federation takes a similar position to that of most haematology specialists in the UK. Clinical opinion in the UK, taken overall, remains relatively cautious, although it is likely that the Cochrane systematic review, and possibly the results of the HTA review, will go some way to increasing acceptance. It is likely that there will be increased pressure for large-scale randomised control trials in the UK.

Users and expertise: Health professionals, patients, citizens

Usership

In the UK in 2007, the number of self-monitoring coagulometer users is believed to be around 12,500, having increased from 8–9,000 at the turn of the century. It is clear that the range of knowledge and expertise associated with the use of coagulometers is extensive, regardless of whether one is a health professional or a patient. Unlike some distance technologies OAT patient self-monitoring (PSM) places a high responsibility on the individual/patient/carer/family. Anticoagulation is high-risk for patients and its monitoring has important implications for self-identity, everyday routines and anxiety about health status. The use of coagulometer technology has to be considered together with knowledge and experience of blood thinning therapy. Thus people's attitudes to and beliefs about warfarin have to be taken into account. For example, in the UK:

> A British Heart Foundation nurse summed up the fears of some of her patients: 'Warfarin is difficult to take. Monitoring is a problem, having to queue for the phlebotomist and wait for the doctor. People are frightened about the risk of bleeding and the lack of information. They talk about warfarin in terms of rat poison. It has a bad image'.
> (saferhealthcare.org.uk, 2006)[4]

As illustrated by the description of warfarin and the INR method above, a working knowledge of the behaviour of blood and anticoagulation therapy sufficient for self-monitoring requires more than everyday lay knowledge. Use of the device demands more than its mechanical operation. I discuss questions of training for self-monitoring below, but mention here just one challenge – knowledge of the strength of the medication: a study from Hong Kong in 2003 found that fewer than half of a sample of patients may understand the strength of the medication, the reason for taking them, or the effect on their body (Tang et al., 2003).

Given the individually defined normal range of INR, it is common for users to understand the INR readings in terms of 'high days' and 'low days' (Hambidge, 2002), 'above-average', 'below-average' and so on. Readings outside these ranges are a cause for concern, but, equally, the more infrequent readings associated with the clinic-based system might be artificially high or low for various reasons, such as a drug interaction where the user is taking more than one form of medication, or where interaction with food substances might occur.

Users of coagulometers for self-management clearly require a degree of 'discipline' in approaching the task of monitoring their INR level. This is shown graphically by one user, following heart surgery:

> Data accumulated from June 2000 to April 2005 contains 263 INR tests which is equal to a frequency of one test per week. Of the 263 INR tests recorded 227 of these tests were within a therapeutic range of 2.50 to 3.50. This is an 86.3% success rate over five years. This is a direct result of frequency of testing.
>
> (Kelman, 2007)

The example illustrates not only a rigorous involvement in record-keeping over an extended period of time but also a commitment to frequent testing, a position that is commonly espoused by committed self-monitoring users, but is controversial among clinicians.

Coagulometer users may develop detailed personal theories ('lay aetiology') about their condition and how they believe monitoring interacts with daily life. For example, another patient, 65 years old and following two DVTs, noted that

> I have recently found that if I have had a stomach upset either from eating rich food, or from a curry or Chinese dish, my INR seems to rise dramatically ... when staying with a family in Peru, before I had the portable device, we were fed rice and mashed potato topped by half a guinea pig; no vegetables or fruit. My INR rose alarmingly.

This user, in fact, had written to *The Lancet* with her account. Another user, living with an artificial heart valve, felt certain that 'stress' was important:

> One of the main things that has a definite but unpredictable effect on the stability of the warfarin level is stress. The effect of the warfarin can be reduced very quickly in a stressful situation, this isn't something

you get told, but when I mentioned it to the pharmacist at the anti-coagulation clinic he admitted that they were aware of that.

(from 'Michael's story', saferhealthcare.org, 2006)

It is clear in the UK that local policies and beliefs among health professionals affect the likelihood that would-be self-monitors will be supported or not. A user associated with *Anticoagulation Europe*, 23 years old, struggled to persuade his anticoagulation clinic of the safety of self-monitoring while away from home travelling in Australia: 'After talking to ACE I re-contacted my clinic and consultants and said that I would self-test and self-dose. The Nurse specialist at the Heart hospital supported me in this action and managed to secure me a secondary back up, whilst I was away. I would email every INR reading and new dose' (Crompton in ACE, 2007). Advocacy tends to emphasise the freedom afforded by the technology, for example ACE presents narratives – and pictures – from patients who recount their experience of using the device while on holiday in far-flung parts of the world (Figure 7.2).

A small local scheme in Wales, UK, included some qualitative evaluation of 16 patients' response to a newly-instituted self-monitoring service. Comments included: 'Self dosing chart would be most helpful; Really improved my life, eliminated 30 mile trip to hospital; Support of Thrombosis Specialist Nurse more than adequate, makes system worthwhile; More control over INR, it is the best thing that has happened to me' (Hughes-Jones, 2006). Patient satisfaction research in this field, given the known methodological and theoretical shortcomings of many such studies, tends to support the acceptability of the technique and arrangements over clinic-based models. Many of these indicative studies are attached to clinical trials (Cromheecke et al., 2000). In this questionnaire study scores for general treatment satisfaction and self-efficacy were (statistically) significantly higher in the self-management group, whereas scores for daily anxieties, distress and strain were significantly lower.

Acceptability to patients of self-monitoring was assessed by questionnaire in a randomised trial study by Gardiner and colleagues, from the UK's Device Evaluation Centre (Gardiner et al., 2005); the study was funded by the MHRA and an educational grant from Roche Diagnostics. The findings from 31 patients who were still self-testing after 3 months were that: the majority of the patients initially found it difficult to obtain an adequate sample, but most subsequently found self-testing easy (55 per cent) or quite easy (32 per cent). Most patients found that they occasionally had to repeat tests. Most patients (87 per cent) were confident in the result that they obtained. Of those with a preference,

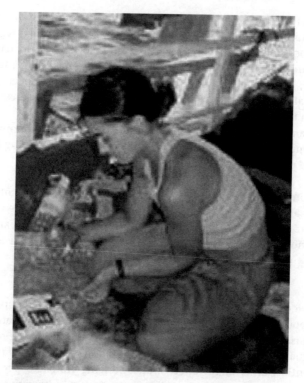

Figure 7.2 A coagulometer user on holiday in Thailand

77 per cent preferred self-testing to clinic. The sample was biased: patients invited to take part in the study were already 'good compliers' with the clinic regime (Gardiner et al., 2005).

There is no formal training programme within the NHS in the UK at the time of writing, though Fitzmaurice has developed a local pilot scheme (and a 'Birmingham model' of primary care based service). This comprises two three-hour sessions covering both practical and theoretical aspects, including quality assurance, which is felt to be sufficient for the majority of patients.

The device manufacturers provide online support services for users, and claim, for example, 'coagulation-monitoring systems tailored to your convenience' and a better clinical outcome: 'testing more frequently means less risks of over- or under-dosing' (Roche Diagnostics, 2006). Training, whether provided by clinical centres or by device manufacturers may address aspects including practical facility in manipulating the equipment; understanding of the INR ratio and its interpretation; vitamin K content of the diet; blood clotting; regularity and responsibility in testing, recording on a log-sheet and reporting results. In some organisational configurations the medical centre may, in effect, be a telemedical 'call centre' with, for example, specialist cardiological staffing. Some training packages attempt to address themselves to the public image of anticoagulation therapy and presumed lay understandings of the medical condition, treatment and monitoring. For example, one of the centres in Germany providing training courses direct to patients suggests these 'theoretical' concerns:

> it is important to eliminate existing prejudices such as 'anticoagulants are rat poisons', 'if I take anticoagulants and get injured, I must die from bleeding', 'on anticoagulation therapy I can't eat anything anymore', 'by the use of anticoagulants one becomes an artificial hemophiliac'.
>
> (Koertke et al. 2005)

Users' views about self-monitoring are indicated partly by reported rates of dropout of schemes and studies. Dropout ('attrition') rates from randomised trials reported internationally have recently been reviewed (Heneghan et al., 2007). The authors report a dropout rate from intervention arms of reviewed studies ranging from 0.0 per cent to 42 per cent. A wide range of possible reasons for withdrawing from self-monitoring was noted. These included: visual impairment, death, preference for general practitioner, distance to travel/non-attendance, difficulty with device including manual dexterity, stopping warfarin therapy and lack of physician support. The authors noted that many patients who self-monitored already had experience of an alternative approach to managing their condition, and might have been inclined to that system.

Patient advocacy

Patient advocacy groups such as the BCPA and ACE are prominent in promoting PSM (ACE 2007), linking with manufacturers and clinician-champions, raising funds to purchase coagulometers for individuals, and negotiating on policy issues. ACE is self-consciously aligned with the 'expert patient' movement in the UK (see section above on policy and governance), and has had some success in negotiating for the testing strips (required to use the coagulometer device) to be made available on prescription through the NHS, from 2002. Patients may also be involved in advising manufacturers; relations between manufacturers and patient advocacy organisations appear quite strong. However, ACE reports receiving many complaints because Primary Care Trusts (PCTs) have been refusing to let GPs prescribe them. ACE has produced a resource pack for patients to try to reverse these decisions. This pack includes, for example, a letter from the Director of ACE addressed to PCTs, which cites several sources of evidence and opinion that support self-monitoring (such as those mentioned in this chapter – Heneghan review, MHRA guidance, Fitzmaurice, NICE guidance on atrial fibrillation and Department of Health expert patient programme and self-care policy), while urging the PCT to re-consider funding of the strips.

Challenging healthcare practice

Many different health professions have an interest in anticoagulation therapy, and it is embedded in the therapeutic and monitoring practices of a variety of different medical conditions. The traditional service model for managing such patients once stabilised has been periodic visits to consultant haematology clinics and interpretation of tests in pathology laboratories. This model is obviously challenged by devolved models of care. Patient self-monitoring is seen by some clinicians to be the next step (Beyth 2005). Assessment of effectiveness and cost-effectiveness of models utilising near-patient point-of-care testing and non-consultant expertise in primary care is growing – although the evidence base has been regarded as small (Murray et al., 2004).

Self-monitoring patients, as noted above, are encouraged to measure their INR much more frequently than would occur with routine clinic visits, a practice which some clinicians question. Fitzmaurice reported that this was a striking feature: 'Testing is recommended every three to seven days, and more often if control of the INR starts to fluctuate. This frequency of testing would be extremely costly, and it is not clear why it is required. In contrast, stable patients in the clinic setting may be tested at intervals of only 10–13 weeks' (Fitzmaurice and Machin, 2001).

One local scheme in the UK was started in the early 2000s on the basis of advertising in the media and demand from patients (Hughes-Jones, 2007). The service reports a steady increase in patients. The service is supported by a locally developed professional guideline. This guideline, interestingly, contains measures that might avoid certain points of controversy in adoption of the technology into routine practice. For example, patients must be 'accessible by telephone' as a condition of embarking on self-monitoring, and 'only patients considered competent to follow total quality management procedures should complete training', and with regard to the controversial issue of frequency of INR testing, the guideline states that

> Blood tests should only be taken at the agreed date and should not be taken out of hours, weekends and bank holidays when there is no TSN (thrombosis specialist nurse) cover, but should the patient feel unwell during these times an INR can be taken prior to taking advice from out of hours medical personnel.
> (Hughes-Jones 2006, NHS Trust 2006)

Such a regime, allied to a requirement for three-monthly review in the clinic, clearly implies a closer communications linkage and specialist-centred control than is envisaged in some models of the coagulometer-based self-testing approach.

The dynamics of coagulometer innovation and governance

A wide range of stakeholders are active in the field of anticoagulation, as illustrated in this case study, and a wide range of evidence from various methodologies, with various forms and forums of presentation, is being constructed. New entrants offering the device in the commercial marketplace and the very recently increasing level of HTA systematic review of clinical and other studies, suggests that the level of attention among policymakers will increase and that there will be increasing pressure on cautious healthcare policy such as that of the UK.

Professional medical associations are cautiously supportive about self-monitoring, but the small-scale innovation that is evident is linked to particular clinical centres where clinical innovators have developed a special interest. Overview of the clinical evidence on the performance of the technology and its potential and actual users suggests that the slow uptake is due not only to the scientific evidence base. Clinical and HTA evidence has been produced at a low level. While the UK Department of Health has recognised the possibilities of self-monitoring, it has been more concerned with possible devolvement of monitoring to primary care, partly because a larger population is involved[5].

As we have seen, coagulometer-assisted self-monitoring and self-management has its champions among clinicians, patient advocacy groups and manufacturers. This is a field where industry and voluntary organisations are clearly powerful drivers, having some limited success in influencing healthcare policy. It is clear also that in the UK there is a divergence of opinion about the evidence of effectiveness of self-monitoring among clinicians and a divergence of medical specialists' attitudes towards experimental schemes to introduce self-monitoring, no doubt partly for reasons of possible resource implications. Evidence about cost-effectiveness is lacking. Likewise, implications for patients, including quality of life, have yet to be properly explored though qualitative research. Thus the limited credibility and fragmentation of the healthcare science in this field are acting to support the conservative position of the healthcare state.

It is clear that the specialist medical professions, especially those in haematology, are reluctant to cede control over many aspects of their conventional expertise and practice. In this respect, the political role of the discourse of 'quality control', evident here in examples from British and Italian professional organisations, is part of a professional project of the expert haematology community to retain control over an institutionalised form of standard-setting. The technical nature of this knowledge, and its embedding in the professional domain of haematology, gives it a social position far distant from the knowledge that even an informed citizen engaged in anticoagulation self-monitoring might readily access. In their key article, which I have cited at several points in this chapter, Fitzmaurice and Machin, writing on behalf of the British Society of Haematology Task Force for Haemostasis and Thrombosis (2001) made this statement about quality control:

> The most widespread British quality control scheme for anticoagulation ... sends freeze dried samples of blood to laboratories every three months. The laboratories reconstitute the freeze dried samples and estimate the international normalised ratio, which is unknown to them ... the performance is expressed as being within or outside a predetermined range around the median INR value obtained by the participants. This process is costly and time consuming for patients, without even taking into consideration the potential difficulties that the patients encounter in reconstituting freeze dried samples. Until data from British trials regarding quality control are available, recommendations can only be based on consensus.
>
> (Fitzmaurice and Machin, 2001)

The juxtaposition in this account of the standardised and specialised procedures of haematological quality control with the potential cost, time and difficulty for patients is indicative of the boundary-drawing typical of many professions that engage in the discursive patrolling and reinforcement of their knowledge base and practices (Freidson, 1986). Unusually, the worlds of technical quality control and the world of patient/user experience are drawn into the same frame in this account.

The state's possible role in citizen training for self-monitoring is contentious. Fitzmaurice and Machin (2001) state that 'it is difficult to know whether training of a similar intensity (i.e. to that offered in Germany) is necessary in the United Kingdom, whether it could be provided within the British NHS, or whether private medical insurance companies would accept the costs ... Further considerations are the 'need for patient consent and the formulation of a contract between the trainer and patient' (op. cit., 2001).

As I have noted, the amount of scientific research, social or otherwise, that examines the citizen-patient's perspective in this field is very small. Questionnaire-based surveys of aggregate 'acceptability' give a very different picture to the one to be gained from individual patient experience. Social acceptability of the technology has been defined more by criteria concerned with competence in using the device such as 'confidence', continued use and evaluation of ease/difficulty, whereas the glimpses of users' accounts, limited as they are, display a richer range of experience and concern about the meaning of INR levels, the embedding of INR measurement in everyday life and lifestyles, and the vagaries of communication with health professionals and their clinical policies. It is, therefore, difficult to construct a credible research-based picture of the 'acceptability' of this technology and its usage in everyday life and healthcare practice. What is known is that it is clear that coagulometer users in the UK, outside of clinical trials at least, are a highly self-selecting set of citizens. Citizen-patients choose to make use of the technology. This raises various questions about the socioeconomic profile of potential users of the technology and 'difficult-to-reach' populations of potential users.

In the absence of NHS recognition, it is likely that a device manufacturer will seek informal means of promoting its devices. A number of linkages between active stakeholders internationally can be discerned. Most conspicuous are links between patient groups and manufacturers. An ISMAAP meeting, 'Living with anticoagulants – dedicated to the exchange of experience between patients' was promoted as the first time a patient's organisation had actively participated in a World Congress of Cardiology, in 2006. Many European countries have a patients' organisation affiliated to ISMAAP. Alliances exist also between clinical champions and device companies.

The healthcare science in this field shows a bias towards self-monitoring supported by regular hospital or clinic checks. An alternative model is for patients to administer their own warfarin *without* self-testing of INR. At least one multi-centre study, undertaken in Italy (Cosmi et al., 2000), suggested that patients could successfully adjust their dose without 'specific training'. This model of partial self-management might appeal to authorities that wish to retain control over the monitoring process.

There are a number of areas of controversy around the innovation of this technology into the healthcare system. In the UK, several of these were summarised by a consultant psychiatrist in the *British Medical Journal*, responding to a negative article. A user of self-monitoring technology himself, he provides 'lay-expert' qualitative insights on issues concerning the financial or other motives for using the technology, the value of frequent testing and the efficiency of standard UK provision compared to other countries:

> Firstly, the suggestion that patient demand for self management is 'partly fuelled by a national media advertising campaign ... (for CoaguChek)' is disingenuous. I wonder how much of an NHS hospital trust haematology department budget is derived from patients attending their Warfarin Clinic? Secondly, it may be that 'routine performance within anti-coagulation clinics in the UK compares favourably with that in other countries', but at what hidden costs to the patients? As I have recently noted ... attending my local hospital Warfarin Clinic every 2 to 3 weeks would occupy 150 working days over 25 years ... Thirdly, 'testing is recommended every 3 to 7 days ... and it is not clear why it is required'. For the first week of my using Coaguchek in August 1997 I measured my INR twice daily ... on at least 10 occasions since then the INR has been 3.1 or higher, and on at least 2 occasions 2.0 or lower from the same medication regime ... If I had attended hospital Warfarin Clinics on the 'low days' my dose of Warfarin would probably have been increased and not re-measured for at least a week, with what consequences? I have already had one major epistaxes [nosebleed] ... urgent ENT surgery, a week in hospital, and a month off work. All secondary to a Warfarin Clinic created INR of 4.8.
>
> (Hambidge, 2002)

So this user has been confident enough to design his own monitoring regime. His letter shows a strong tension between the possibilities of a

'DIY' approach to using the device in the context of his medical condition and the perceived constraints and possible failures that he sees as inherent in the traditional clinic-based regime.

Regulatory agencies in the UK have been directly involved in commissioning and undertaking safety and performance evaluations, beyond the requirements of the *In Vitro* MDD. Surprisingly perhaps, although the UK's NPSA has examined anticoagulation, it has not examined self-monitoring. It is difficult to judge the relative salience of the different scientific evidence that has been produced around this technology. In fact, a *lack* of evidence, especially in the area of cost-effectiveness is probably the most significant feature of the evidential landscape here. The calls for large multi-centre randomised trials act as a rein even on enthusiastic clinicians and local policymakers. At the same time, there have been a number of shifts in the organisation of regulatory agencies that affect the regulatory evidentiality of point-of-care devices. The MHRA in the UK has responsibility for the safety of POCT coagulometers, but has recently decided no longer to perform technical testing themselves, leaving them with responsibility for investigating reported adverse incidents under the vigilance system. It appears that the regulatory and evaluatory agencies concerned entertain diverging criteria of assessment – for example, the NHS CEP taking the position that 'CE marked IVDs are fit for purpose, unless proven otherwise, so testing is not required' (Gardiner, personal communication 2007). Such a position draws a boundary around the evidential standards for placing on the market, sufficient for national-level purchasing policy, but excluding specific evaluation of patient safety.

Coagulometer technology and society

It is clear that the language of 'monitoring' and 'management', associated with the care of people with chronic medical conditions, is the language of healthcare provision and medicine. Although the coagulometer, and the knowledge and expertise involved in its use, provide the opportunity for some individual autonomy and separation from regimes of dependence on healthcare systems, the fact that coagulometer users and advocates also use the language of self-monitoring suggests that adoption of the technology amounts to a form of medicalisation. However, this is not medicalisation as traditionally understood, as the progressive encroachment of institutionalised medical epistemologies into everyday life. Rather, and especially because of the key involvement of the commercial private sector, it is closer to the 'biomedicalization' proposed by Clarke and colleagues in the US, in which the interests of medicine and 'technoscience' are increasingly drawn together in ways that shape the semantic environment in which as citizens we negotiate our personal identities in and around patienthood (Clarke et al., 2003).

Users of coagulometers may identify ambiguously with the status of patienthood. Many are able perhaps to alleviate the dependency implied in this status – ironically – through use of these high-tech devices. Arguably, however, clinic attenders may be less medicalised through the monitoring process than people who have a monitoring device always at hand, in a similar way to a mobile phone. In the case of the UK it is interesting to consider the implications of the fact that (at present) the devices are not available through the publicly funded NHS. Users have to purchase the devices directly (though in some cases they are funded through charitable donation or fundraising). Therefore, the technology has the marketplace status of a consumer product. It may be that although this clearly limits the social range from which the majority of users are likely to come, and thus inequities in access are likely to remain, there may be some psychological reward and contribution to motivation and self-concept that this structural circumstance promotes. In summary, the configuring of coagulometer users may be as much due to the socioeconomic circumstance of the diffusion routes of the device as to the qualities of the device itself and the care milieu. As the advocacy activity around the device shows, these features of the world of anticoagulating citizens are themselves the subject of stakeholder representations.

Research to compare the 'meaning' of coagulometer use under different socioeconomic conditions, such as those in Germany and the UK, has yet to be undertaken. Such research holds the potential to shed light upon the extent to which the possible experience of autonomy associated with the device is attributable to the informed use of the device itself, or also to the societal or market conditions under which it is obtained or provided. The experience of 'domesticating' the coagulometer and the psychosocial implications of coagulometer use thus constitute major gaps in the current (qualitative) research record in anticoagulation therapy, unlike the PSA test described in Chapter 5.

The process of interpretation of test results is beginning to be acknowledged as possibly undertaken safely and routinely by self-monitoring patients, using the same standardised measurement system as used by clinical specialists. Given that home-testing kits for PSA levels are available in the marketplace, it may be revealing to ask why the self-testing issue has become quite widely examined in the world of anticoagulation but not in the world of prostate cancer detection. The reason may lie in the difference in the healthcare and medical contexts. With anticoagulation, there is an established therapy, whose effects can be gauged through a single method of measurement. The interpretative link between test results and therapy is thus simple, linear and stable. With the PSA test on the other hand, although this also is situated medically in the context of life-threatening conditions, for any non-normal test result the interpretation and any advisable therapy is beset with uncertainties, and the interpretative link is thus multi-linear and highly insecure, as described in the case study in this book. The expertise required to be a 'competent user' of these two self-testing technologies is thus very different in nature.

One of the key threads running through this book is the dynamics of the relationships between technologies and their users, and the direction and nature of any 'shaping' that might take place. This chapter has shown that coagulometer users show a degree of autonomy and inventiveness in operating and interpreting the device and its outputs in everyday life (one might of course make the same observation about, say, driving motor cars or bicycle-riding). End-users appear to have little influence in shaping the design features of the device itself. While the organisation and design of the device cannot be altered by the user (or, at least, it is very difficult to envisage an alternative use parallel to the way that the gramophone record turntable became re-envisaged as a musical instrument for a new form of DJ (Pinch, 2003)), it is clear that there are features of its use with which the user is able and often willing to be creative. Most obviously, users may control the frequency of testing, and consequently may decide on adjustments of therapy – though within the limits of a narrow therapeutic range. There appear to be no instances of coagulometers being used entirely outside the auspices of a formal healthcare regime of some sort, as one might expect (though evidence of this would be better established than assumed). The devices are inoperable without a set of part-generic, part-individualised knowledge about application of the technology in the life of particular patients. Thus there is evidence of inventiveness, flexibility and self-determination in its actual deployment. Equally, there is evidence of a wide variety of possible regimes of care constructed by healthcare providers.

The use of coagulometer technology is not determined only by its physical design and its development trajectory. Prospective users enter upon a course of socialisation into use of the device. Part of this process is structured training programmes, but part is a development and application of personal experience that includes personal understandings and assessments of, for example, the interaction of diet and test results. Coagulometer use is the outcome of a variable mixture of designer-conceived technology, manufacturers' training, clinical conventions, practices and rules adapted for the device, and users' own theories and practices, which might include interaction with carers or patient support/advocacy groups. Unlike the other device technologies discussed in this book, the coagulometer may become involved in processes of literal domestication (Silverstone and Haddon, 1996) in which users, seen here as citizen-patients, involved in complex sets of social and medical relationships, 'appropriate' technologies and the associated healthcare system interactions into their everyday life.

However, a focus on domestication and similar concepts runs the risk of overlooking the upstream politics and economics of device innovation. One of the starting-points for the approach to analysis in this book is the alleged lack of attention (in Science and Technology Studies analysis) to the role of the state in configuring users (Rose and Blume 2003). There is clear evidence of actions of the healthcare state in steering the diffusion of coagulometers, both through the NHS and through the evidence-marshalling by national-level HTA and other agencies. The healthcare state also has exercised a shaping influence via the variable clinical guidance constructed and promulgated by local anticoagulation professional communities and centres. Compared to the other case studies discussed in this book, the state's role in the dynamics of shaping coagulometer users has not been far-reaching. In state-endorsed evidentiality, discourse about cost, patients' expertise and self-monitoring practices are key points of tension in the innovation pathway of anti coagulation self-monitoring.

The clinical world of anticoagulation is inhabited by a wide range of medical specialties – cardiology and cardiac surgery, cardiothoracic surgery, haematology, primary care, specialist thrombosis nursing, stroke specialists and so on. This very diversity of clinical ownership of anticoagulation services may itself be a factor impeding the development of self-monitoring in the UK, because of the difficulty of achieving policy coordination across the range of disciplines.

Overall, therefore, the innovation pathway around coagulometers for self-monitoring can be characterised by governance in which local and national agencies of the healthcare state are strong. In terms of political economy in the UK the technology is ambiguous because it is located partly inside the public healthcare system and partly, more strongly, inside the private consumer goods sector. While assumptions of individual autonomy may be inscribed into the device itself 'by design', the healthcare system and regulatory governance embed into the user-ship of the technology institutionalised practices of expert medical authority and care. Assertive or favoured patients can shape themselves as active, autonomous citizens, but the nature of this experience in terms of quality of life is not yet explored through research. Coagulometer users may be regarded as being involved in processes of co-construction in which aspects of society are designed into the technology, and society – in the form of healthcare practice and evidentiality – configures the possibilities of its usership.

8
Device or Drug? Governation of Tissue Engineering

Introduction

The definition of the borderlines of technologies is important to society, to science and to political economies. There have been examples of technologies that are developed beyond discrete material boundaries in the previous case studies in this book. Implantable hip prostheses gain bioactive coatings, infusion pumps become information and communication technologies, creating a new type of healthcare product. Classification systems and processes are fundamental to anthropological understandings of society, and become deeply embedded in the structuring of the industrial economy and in medical practice (Bowker and Star, 2000). Boundaries are 'necessary for making meanings ... [and] ... have real material consequences' (Barad, 1998: 187). The subverting character of contemporary biotechnology means that such socio-material boundaries have to be regarded as plastic. The re-drawing of these boundaries is part of processes of re-ordering societies' institutions, cognitive and practice domains and moralities. The negotiation of technology's borderlines may or may not align closely with classifications of contemporary industrial sectors, which are crucial to industrial and economic policymaking. Regulatory governance and technical standardisation processes interact with the shaping of new sectors or sub-sectors. Commercial and public funders orient themselves to sectorally defined arenas of industrial and technological innovation.

In this book, the technologies discussed so far have been identifiable quite unproblematically as medical device technologies, products of a medical device industry, albeit a sector organised around sub-sectors such as diagnostics, equipment and surgical implants. Not all medical technology innovations fall neatly into this sort of categorisation.

159

Especially troubling to such institutionalised classifications is the current avalanche of biological and gene-related developments. In this final case study chapter, therefore, I consider the development of the complex field of the so-called 'tissue-engineering' technologies, which challenge existing borderlines – industrial, scientific, clinical and regulatory. Tissue engineering (TE) has been debated, though not as widely in the public sphere as one might have expected, as a key strand of the much-heralded and much-hyped regenerative medicine of the future.

TE technologies are difficult to define. Indeed, this chapter will treat the societal definition of TE as a topic in itself. TE technologies typically, though not always, combine manufactured biomaterials with living, viable human tissues or cells. The ambiguity of definitions has been crucial to the development of regulatory activity that has attempted to map a clear 'technological zone' (Barry, 2001) for tissue engineering[1]. Some TE technologies are already in clinical use, others are under development. The development of the field has been and continues to be the subject of much speculation and uncertainty. The development of products and their distribution into healthcare has been modest. There have been some commercial failures, and scientific and industrial participants in the field feel that it suffers from an 'image problem'. The technology has been promoted by industrial policymakers, clinical and scientific researchers and by manufacturers. Examination of the development and diffusion of TE products/services at this early stage requires an examination of the active stakeholder constituencies, in this case in particular the interaction of regulators and industry.

The 'deviceness' of TE products has been a notion contested in regulatory debate. Such technologies have a peculiar status within formal regulatory frameworks, their typically hybrid material composition disturbing established categories of medical device and pharmaceutical regulations (Abraham and Lewis, 2000). The technical ambiguity and hybridity of TE is useful in revealing the processes by which actors attempt to promote particular versions of TE as a regulatable technology, under conditions of evidential uncertainty.

This case study presents a new variation in comparison to those previously discussed. By investigating an unstable technology, still 'under construction', we have the opportunity of examining the sorts of politico-economic processes that define the contours shaping the pathway of new technologies from scientific development into societal practice. The plural 'assessment' of TE technologies combines assessment not only of safety and efficacy/effectiveness, which have been prominent in the other case studies in this book, but also assessment criteria conventionally deemed social and ethical. Such 'social' and/or 'ethical' issues may be raised in the case of TE especially because of concerns about the sourcing and processing of tissues and cells, and because of the use of animal materials and links in some cases to human embryonic stem cell and human-animal hybrid research.

The chapter draws on extensive empirical research in the UK and EU[2]. Because it examines the regulatory aspects of TE technology, it has a focus primarily on the EU negotiations of new regulation, rather than the UK focus that the previous case studies have adopted. The chapter considers the history of TE, pointing to the socio-political process of its regulation. It makes the case that regulation is as much a process of socio-technical innovation as it is a process of control and surveillance. Much of the shaping of the TE zone can be shown through the discourses which stakeholders deployed in attempting to negotiate a new regulatory regime. I analyse the formation of a new regime as a constructive process which defines the terrain and the rules of engagement for tissue-engineered things to come. In order to capture the regulatory ordering of a TE zone, I propose the concept of 'governation' to suggest the mixture of *govern*ance and innov*ation* to be observed in the process of regulatory policymaking.

Tissue engineering technology and the marketplace

TE was first conceived in the mid 1980s in the US, and credit for defining the field, in the advanced western countries at least, is traced to an article in *Science* by scientists from Boston (Langer and Vacanti, 1993). TE combines aspects of medicine, cell and molecular biology, materials science and engineering. The material production and constitution of TE technologies is very diverse. One influential definition – from a Europe-level scientific advisory body – describes TE as the 'regeneration of biological tissue through the use of cells, with the aid of supporting structures and/or biomolecules' (SCMPMD, 2001). The materials involved in TE include viable human cells or tissue, growth factors to stimulate cell activity and cell culture materials such as human serum, bovine and/or murine (mouse) cells. Some products have a base layer of collagen (fibrous material) which can be human or bovine. Manufactured biomaterials are often also included, e.g. polymer micro-scaffolds to provide a suitable physical structure on which live cells may proliferate. A key distinction is whether products are made using a patient's own cells for auto-therapy of the same patient ('autologous', i.e. a customised product or service such as knee cartilage implantation

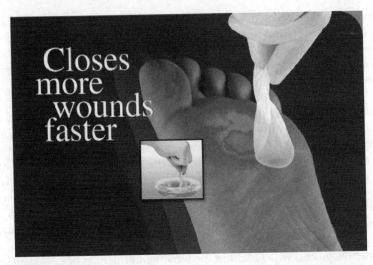

Figure 8.1   Apligraf: a 'skin equivalent' containing viable human donor cells

noted above) or whether multiple donors/patients are involved ('allogeneic' – i.e. off-the-shelf product such as skin systems for burns).

The two main types of TE application already in clinical practice are cartilage repair for traumatic injury to the articular cartilage of the knee ('Autologous Cartilage Implantation' – ACI) and skin systems for burns and chronic ulcers, especially those associated with diabetes (Figure 8.1). Other current applications include bone substitutes. Future developments, some of which have been subject to clinical trial, are expected to include vascular prostheses, bladder constructs, organ-assist devices (liver, kidney), whole organs, structures (heart valves, cardiac tissue to repair heart muscle following heart attack, joints), neurological tissues and stem cell therapies. Whether the latter should be included inside the boundary of the TE zone has been much debated (this point is discussed below under Policy/Governance).

A leading American commentator on the industry of TE has described its trajectory as a roller coaster comprising: '1995–2000 – Years of fat; 2001–2003 – The perfect storm; 2004 onward – Sadder, wiser, poorer ... but remarkably robust' (Lysaght, 2006). It is clear that there was an early period of expansion in which private and public investment was high, followed by a period of retrenchment in which clinical trials failed and new products failed to be adopted (Lysaght and Hazlehurst, 2004), followed by a re-orientation which is continuing. Lysaght summarised the early, problematic history as being due to a 'better mousetrap' mentality: limited improvements over existing therapies together with high manufacturing costs, high cost of regulatory approval, weak marketing and firms lacking clear reimbursement strategies (op. cit., 2006). The costs of individual applications are relatively high and therefore need to be justified. Reimbursement of costs by state authorities has been a contentious issue internationally, and according to some analysts this was the main reason for the bankruptcy of early US firms such as Advanced Tissue Sciences and Organogenesis. A number of products were abandoned at the stage of clinical trial in the US, including bioartificial liver products, an aid to coronary artery graft patency and a bladder product for adult incontinence.

TE is supported by government public funding. For example, in the UK research councils have provided funds for academic and commercial networks such as REMEDI and a national TE scientific research collaboration. The EC has supported cross-national networks such as a €25 million STEPS programme (Systems Approach to Tissue Engineering Processes and Products), a 25-partner 13-country consortium addressing manufacturing and production issues and led by the University of Liverpool, UK, Fidia, one of Italy's leading TE companies and the 'ScanBalt Regenerative Medicine Knowledge Network', a north-European knowledge region including TE, dedicated to research, development and education.

Estimates of the market for tissue engineered products have varied widely over the last few years. The largest market would be the US with estimates for skin systems of approximately US$ 20 million in 2003, and some expectations that it could grow to US$190 million by 2005. The EU market for tissue engineered products was estimated to be €50–100 million, and significant growth is expected (Schutte, 2003). The EC itself commissioned the most exhaustive publicly available study of the state of the market in Europe to date as part of the development of proposals for new regulation. This was produced through its own research facility, the Joint Research Centre – Institute for Prospective Technological Studies (IPTS). Some of the key findings were:

- Low level of activity, mainly technology-intensive biotech SMEs
- A few big pharmaceutical and medical device companies
- Approximately 113 companies in Europe in 2003 – leaders being Germany, UK, France, Sweden
- 35 products on EU market in 2003 – 18 skin, 15 cartilage, 2 bone
- 44 new products planned to market 2004–8, of which 30 autologous
- Market projections varying wildly
- Some company failures and restructuring

- Some diversification into testing as well as or instead of therapeutic products
- Many of the 'TE' companies moving to work with stem cells
- No single product available in all EU countries
- Bias toward autologous products in Europe
- Lack of data available on hospital-based tissue engineering work.

(summarised from Bock et al., 2003)

In general the TE field can be characterised as beset by a large number of uncertainties which inhibit growth and stabilisation. Factors underlying this uncertainty include: the multidisciplinary science; potential markets and reimbursement issues; business models; production models (automation and 'scale-up' issues); safety and efficacy, and the forms of evidence required or appropriate; ethics – for example, commodification; consent, ownership, traceability of donors and surveillance of recipients; animal material; and definitions of 'Tissue Engineering' itself. TE may or may not be on the point of achieving significant stability (Lysaght, 2006). Lysaght estimated in 2006 that over 150 'small Tissue Engineering/Regenerative Medicine firms' were active in the US, Europe and Asia, and noted that several major companies had committed major development programmes – Johnson & Johnson, Genzyme and Medtronic – the latter, interestingly from the perspective of this book, primarily a medical device company. On the other hand, one can point to the withdrawal by Smith & Nephew in 2006 from its tissue engineered wound care business, which was taken over by US companies.

Turning to EC negotiation of a new regulatory framework for TE, companies in the late 1990s to early 2000s were faced with separate national authorities with different regimes or no regime at all applied to marketing authorisation for TE products. Assessing the implications of harmonised EU regulation, the IPTS report concludes that 'the (proposed new) regulation could help build trust in this new technology, thereby encouraging its acceptance in medical practice and reimbursement policies' (Bock et al., 2003). Before considering the development of this new regulatory governance for TE, I first turn to consider the usership of tissue-engineered therapies.

Usership and healthcare science

The users of tissue engineered products may be divided into users of products that are in healthcare practice or in clinical trials and the users that are constructed in promissory, visionary and regulatory scenarios. Here, I consider the direct users of the technology in practice, who are clinicians, primarily surgeons of various specialties depending upon the application, but also some nursing specialists, especially in the case of wound care technologies. From the perspective of the healthcare system, the adoption of these technologies into use depends upon assessment of quality and safety under relevant regulatory regimes and on evaluations of effectiveness and cost-effectiveness, typically accomplished through the clinical and healthcare sciences.

For clinical users a variety of concerns about tissue-engineered products arise, most obviously the evaluation of the safety and effectiveness of the technology in clinical use. Such evaluation is necessarily limited because of the relatively small number of products that have reached clinical application or the trial phase. The relative paucity of evidence about this aspect of the usership of TE technologies, and problems with making a case for cost-effectiveness in publicly funded healthcare systems, are among the reasons why as a technological zone the field has experienced difficulties in achieving a clear identity.

From a clinical perspective, the issue of whether a technology or technical procedure is tissue-engineered *per se* or not, while not irrelevant, is certainly not the primary consideration in considering whether to adopt it. Such decisions are the outcome of complex commercial, evidential and policy gatekeeper activity. The literature reporting on the clinical results and efficacy of tissue engineered technologies is growing, but I do not attempt to review this literature in a systematic or other fashion here. It will be sufficient to give some examples to indicate the issues of clinical usership and healthcare system adoption that arise, the sources of evidence, and the methodologies that have been constructed for producing clinical evidence for TE applications.

Users of wound care TE products have reviewed the scientific evidence about tissue-engineered and other products with a biological action, concluding by the canons of the EBM hierarchy of the strength of research designs that

> Randomised controlled trials are lacking for many biological products, and the current evidence for many biological based treatments is based on non-randomised prospective trials, retrospective reviews, small case series.
>
> (Enoch et al., 2005)

Users of burns technologies have requirements for products used in clinical practice, not least whether they can be manipulated readily as part of surgical procedures:

> Practical and safe transplantation necessitates 'easy to handle' scaffolds that could be fabricated as carriers for the transfer of not only epithelial cells but of dermal elements as well ... The CBSGs (composite biocompatible skin graft) are much easier to handle than the conventional cultured epidermal autografts and are good human skin substitutes in terms of durability, biocompatibility, high seeding efficacy for keratinocytes [skin cells], high graft take rate, and low infection rate.
>
> (Atiyeh et al., 2005)

Cost and familiarity also play a part in the clinician-user's assessment of TE products:

> *Dermagraft*™ is high cost, is high tech and looks the part. *Promogran* is not so high tech but it has a higher cost than a standard dressing but it looks like a dressing.
>
> (Wound care clinician-researcher, interview by author, 2003)

Clinical expertise becomes enmeshed with the technological practices of medical specialties. Alignment between industrial-scientific activity and the world of clinical practice is crucial to the innovation pathways that TE might take. Innovative technologies may be 'disruptive' in the sense of presenting challenges to the existing division of clinical labour and the organisation of medical work. Thus, for example, the new subspecialty of interventional cardiology has arisen worldwide, in association with the development of the new surgical technology. Without percutaneous transluminal coronary angioplasty (PTCA) and stents (manufactured tubes that fit inside arteries) this subspecialty would not exist. Thus it seems likely *a priori* that some TE technologies will be presented with a more receptive and more organisable clinical usership than others. An internationally prominent wound care researcher and academic entrepreneur explained the problems for product acceptance of there being 'no woundcareology', and the power that accrues with recognised medical specialties:

> For the chronic wounds there is this issue that in the UK that most of the chronic wounds are seen by nurses and with the greatest

respect, nurses are not necessarily going to be given that power or budget to actually pay for the expensive tissue engineered thing, it's probably going to be hospital consultants who will control the use of these products ... There again, in probably France and Germany there's also a lot of *medical* input into decision making of what goes on, on chronic wounds.

(Clinician-researcher,
interview by author, 2003)

The emergence of the cross-cutting specialism of Tissue Viability Nursing may counter this view of the structure of professional wound care practice to some extent, and has been credited with promoting the uptake of advanced woundcare products, of which TE products are a subset (DTI, 2005).

Turning to consider usership at the level of the healthcare system, a very modest amount of analysis within the HTA scientific regime has been undertaken. In the case of the knee cartilage procedure (ACI), systematic review has been conducted in the UK. A recent review (updating an earlier one) compared ACI to more established techniques for treating similar conditions, concluding that

There is insufficient evidence at present to say that ACI is cost-effective compared to microfracture or mosaicplasty. Longer-term outcomes are required. In the absence of hard evidence, economic modelling using some assumptions about long-term outcomes ... suggests that ACI would be cost-effective because it is more likely to produce hyaline cartilage, which is more likely to be durable and to prevent osteoarthritis in the longer (e.g. 20 years) term.

(Clar et al., 2004)

The Clar report has formed the basis for guidance issued by NICE, which is discussed below, in the section on policy and governance. HTA of tissue-engineered wound care is cautious. One study showed that while skin system *Apligraf* plus 'good wound care' treatment resulted in 12 per cent reduction in cost over one year compared to good wound care only (Redekop et al., 2003), for TE wound care technology in general there was still weak scientific basis for the cost-effectiveness of TE treatments for skin ulcers (Bock et al., 2003).

Innovative methodological developments in health economics (part of the UK MATCH programme mentioned in Chapter 3) have produced a 'headroom' method that facilitates an assessment of the likely commercial viability of different tissue-engineered innovations in treatment of bladder and urethral conditions. The method was able to distinguish between engineered urethral tissue, which appeared unpromising, and TE for bladder resection in the case of cancer, which appeared to have potential (McAteer et al., 2007).

Tissue engineered products may have implications for the personal identity of its end-users. Colleagues have discussed this issue elsewhere in relation to tissue-engineered autologous cartilage implantation (Kent et al., 2006). It would appear that the implications for 'self' of autologous 'self-repair' technologies such as ACI are very different to that of allogeneic multi-donor technologies where analytic concepts such as biovalue and intercorporeality have much more purchase (cf. Waldby, 2002a, 2002b).

Clinical users and patients may express ethical concerns deriving from cultural or religious beliefs. This has been raised by some clinicians on the basis of their experience with patients as an issue of medical ethics in relation to the animal materials used in many products:

> Currently, consent is not obtained when biological products (including allografts and xenografts) are applied to patients belonging to diverse religious and cultural backgrounds. Furthermore, the awareness of the healthcare professionals about the constituents of biological products has never been evaluated nor whether they have the necessary knowledge to obtain informed consent.
>
> (Enoch et al., 2005)

These clinical authors surveyed 100 health professionals in the UK, specialising in wound care, to assess the extent of knowledge of the materials used in a variety of leading wound dressings. Some of their results are summarised in Table 8.1, showing relatively high proportions of lack of knowledge on this issue

Table 8.1 Percentages of wound care health professionals professing lack of knowledge of the constituents of wound care technologies

Product includes 'pig' or 'cow' biol. material	Application	Per cent of health professionals 'don't know'
Apligraf	Burns, ulcers	68%
Biobrane	biol. dressing	57%
Integra	burns	30%
Alloderm	burns	74%

Source: Based on Enoch et al., 2005.

A number of issues important to clinical usership have been illustrated in this section, including not only issues of practical application, but also clinical organisation and the evidence-base that might influence clinical opinion. Thus the usership of tissue-engineered technologies currently available, varying between regions and between different national healthcare systems, is diverse, depending especially on the nature of particular TE technologies. The users of wound care technologies may include pharmacists, burns specialists, community and specialist nurses, plastic surgeons and dermatologists, among others. Conversely, in the case of cartilage implantation of the knee, the professional usership is much more clearly definable as primarily orthopaedic surgeons, a point that has implications for the innovation pathway into practice. I now turn to consider the role in TE technology innovation of regulatory governance processes in Europe, and here it is interesting to note that among the stakeholders active in regulatory debate 'at EU-level', clinical practitioners are generally regarded as having a relatively weak voice.

Policy and governance

The most active stakeholders in shaping the regulatory regime for tissue-engineered technology have been the industries involved, the national and pan-European regulatory and policymaking agencies and the national governments' health policy constituencies. It is widely accepted that the industries have been the prime movers in seeking new regulation to embrace TE technology. The medical professions have had relatively low direct participation, and patients' and public voices have been conspicuously absent, although a specialist bioethics contribution has been evident. In this section, I outline the main strands in the development of new regulation for TE in the EU, given that this produces legislation that is applicable to member states. I use qualitative empirical research materials in order to illustrate the innovative, technology zone-shaping forces of regulatory regime-building, and the conflicting sectoral and national interests that have struggled to define the societal significance of tissue and cell manipulation.

Boundaries for technological zones

The arrival of TE challenges numerous boundaries of authority and expertise: national/European, medicine/device, human tissue/animal tissue, tissue bank/industry, commerce/public health and the bounded structures and habits of existing regulatory agencies. 'Human Tissue Engineered Product' (hTEP) is one of a range of terms that has been used to describe this group of healthcare products. The absence of agreed terminology within the policy arena indicates both the discursive construction of these objects and their instability. In the early 2000s, over 20 different terms were being considered among regulatory agencies for the designation of products created through TE. These included terms such as biohybrid systems, human-derived therapeutic products and biological devices.

In 2006, US analyst Lysaght, quoted above in reference to the TE market, used a definition of TE as products that 'Combine living cells and biomaterials into a single medical device; Utilize processed living cells as therapeutic or diagnostic reagents; and Create living tissue, in vitro or in vivo, for therapeutic purposes'. He also excludes stem-cell companies which 'lack a strong product development focus'. Notable here is the use of the term 'device' which would be absent from many definitions, and exclusion of stem cell companies. This terminology points to the vexed issues of the interests of different industrial sectors that have been attempting to shape the TE zone. The importance of such classification is illustrated by a UK regulator explaining how the regulatory agency would react if a manufacturer approached them with a new product that might fall into the TE field:

> there are several issues. I mean the most fundamental one is what is the product classification, like you know is it a medicine, is it a device or is it another regulatory category because that's fundamental.
>
> (MHRA official, interview by author, 2006)

From regulatory patchwork to coherent ensemble?

Some TE products before the negotiation of a TE regulatory regime had already been regulated as pharmaceuticals, while some parts of combination products (for example, synthetic scaffolds) needed to gain approval as medical devices. Manufacturers had to satisfy differing national regulations and approaches to these issues across the EU. As officials from the British device regulatory agency stated:

> the same innovative product may be variously regulated as a medical device, a medicinal product, a tissue, a modified organ or a consumer product.
>
> (Cox and Tinkler, 2000)

Tissue engineered technologies sat uneasily in the patchwork of EU regulation during the 1990s and early 2000s. Unlike the other device technologies discussed in this book, they were not (and in some cases continue not to be, as will become clear below) unequivocally classified in the scope of the medical devices regulatory regime. They were often conceived of in regulatory policy communities themselves as 'borderline' or 'hybrid' products – occupying a 'regulatory vacuum' at the borders of existing regulatory frameworks (Faulkner et al., 2003). There are also some products that combine components requiring assessment under more than one regime: 'many tissue engineered products, such as bioartificial organs are combination products in the regulatory sense, that is, they may constitute a combination of a drug, device or biological product' (Hellman, 1997).

Regulatory anomalies

It is worth illustrating the regulatory complexity of some products, because this is important to the sectoral negotiations of new regulation. *Epicel*, for example, produced by biotechnology company Genzyme, was first introduced in 1987. It encapsulates issues of classification and evaluation as a device or a medicine, and in this case, further, whether it is human or animal, alive or dead, inert or animate. Epicel is a treatment for severe extensive burns, for which autografts of a patient's own surviving skin may not be adequate. It is grown from a patient's own skin cells co-cultured with mouse cells to form grafts – autologous, engineered skin. Reportedly, enough skin material can be grown to cover a patient's entire body in 16 days. In the US it was originally classified and approved as a medical device. The prevailing definition of xenotransplantation (animal to human) was confined largely to whole organs, and so possible risks from material such as irradiated mouse cells were not considered by xenotransplant regulatory bodies. Subsequently, a regulatory focus on transpecies disease increased both in the US and in the UK's interim xenotransplantation regulatory authority (UKXIRA). The status of Epicel as a straightforward 'device' then began to be disturbed. Epicel is currently described by its manufacturer Genzyme as an 'autologous cell therapy product' that is 'co-cultured with mouse cells to form cultured epidermal autografts', and uses 'a cell culture medium containing bovine serum' (Genzyme Biosurgery website, www.genzymebiosurgery.com/corp/gzbx_p_ci_index.asp). In EC consultations about future European TE legislation, the issue of possible overlap with the Medical Products Directive (i.e. pharmaceutical) definition of cell therapy medicinal products, and the possibility that some products would be both TE and medicinal, had been raised (EC DG Enterprise, 2002). Thus the ambiguous regulatory identity of Epicel is highlighted here. An industry expert in 'regulatory affairs' explained the inextricable link between the discursive malleability of such a technology and its cellular make-up:

> In principle, products like Epicel should not be regulated under the annexes of 2003/63 (cell therapy medicinal products) because the biological properties of the cells have not been substantially altered as a result of their manipulation. Key question: what is 'significantly altered' and what constitutes 'structurally and functionally analogous' is probably a moot point as the level of regulatory scrutiny is likely to be equal by either path.
>
> (Genzyme official,
> personal communication, 2005)

Even more contentious than Epicel, the skin product *Apligraf*, mentioned above, has achieved the status of a *cause célèbre* among regulatory actors in the EU. This is because, although this was the first TE product to receive regulatory approval anywhere and is now the most successful TE product worldwide in terms of sales, when it was presented to the European regulators for market approval, it proved impossible for them to fit it into any existing regulatory product classification, and they were unable to decide how to assess it. It was neither a medical device, regulatable under the device directive certification system, nor a medicine regulatable under the centralised European Medicines Agency (EMEA) system or by 'mutual recognition' between national authorities. It therefore did not receive marketing approval and could not be distributed in the EU-wide market. In fact, it was approved in some individual countries such as Ireland and Switzerland.

In the face of this complexity, there has been a widely, although not unanimously, perceived need for 'new regulation' for human tissues and TE. The human tissue *engineering* regulation refers to manufacturing and market approval, excluding the accreditation of safety and quality of sourcing and storage covered by the 2004 Tissues and Cells Directive. These two jurisdictions were already separated in the UK, whose regulatory work in the early 2000s included a tightening of standards and accountability through a code of practice for tissue banking (Department of Health, 2001b) and a voluntary code of practice for manufacturers of 'human-derived therapeutic products'

(MDA, 2002b). In these developments the distinction between traditional tissue banking for transplantation and the emerging activity of engineering tissues in implants is increasingly troubled, as tissue banks move to engage in manipulation and industry engages in tissue banking.

Moving from tissues and cells as tradeable commodities in themselves, tissue engineered products have been the subject of regulatory strategy-making which makes the zone or sector-building aim of the regulation very explicit, the aims being:

- High level of health protection
- Harmonise market access, improve functioning of internal market
- Foster competitiveness of European undertakings
- Provide overall legal certainty ... allowing for ... flexibility at technical level.

(EC, 2005:3)

It can be seen here that the primary risks towards which the emerging product regulation is oriented are, first, technological risk to human health, especially the risk of viral transmission due to infected donor materials, and, second, risks to commercial viability and competitiveness. The way in which these risks are framed in policymaking discourse and the relation of this to issues of comparative efficacy of technologies within healthcare systems has been analysed elsewhere (Faulkner et al., 2008).

Finally, the scope and definition of a TE technological zone is influenced by attempts to distinguish it from other potentially overlapping or cognate zones. In the early debates such 'threats' were portrayed as coming from a variety of sources such as embryonic stem cells, cloning, animals and whole organ transplantation:

We should not include organs in this measure on cells and tissues. Organs are for another day. Equally, this is not the time to permit cloned human embryos or hybrid human animal embryos to have their cells and tissues used for transplants.

(MEP Bowis, in European
Parliament, 2003)

Is tissue engineering special?

In the regulatory policy debate on the shape of a TE regulatory body in Europe a number of different models have been proposed. An early recommendation from the high status Scientific Committee for

Medicinal Products and Medical Devices (SCMPMD, 2001) was for a separate free standing Regulatory Authority for TE. At this time TE was frequently framed as falling *between* medical devices and pharmaceutical regimes (Table 8.2). Most prominent in the first phase of consultation and negotiation was the distinction between autologous and allogeneic applications of TE – in other words, an organising principle based on the origin of the starting materials used. Individual self-repair, autologous applications, in a widely shared perception were initially regarded as less risky, especially because of low risk of viral contamination. Not only were they regarded as biologically safe but also were regarded as an 'ethics-free zone', to quote one scientist-informant. In particular, the cartilage regeneration procedure, ACI, was framed by scientists as a 'self-contained' procedure (Kent et al., 2006). In the first phase of the regulatory debate on the proposals for regulation of human TE products (EC DG Enterprise, 2004a; 2004b; 2004c), the autologous/allogeneic principle was used as the hinge on which to hang a two-tier system of regulation, in which allogeneic products would be authorised through a centralised EU regulatory authority and autologous products would be authorised primarily by mutually-recognising national authorities. Thus the difference in material origin was enshrined in an institutional division of labour and responsibility. As the summary of consultation by DG Enterprise reported:

> Autologous vs. allogeneic: the procedural distinction ... was generally considered as a possible starting point, but many contributions stressed that it should be complemented with other relevant criteria. Thus, some respondents proposed to consider parameters relating to the composition of the cell population in the tissue, the physiological function of the tissue or the risk induced by the product in relation to its functionality. Other criteria were proposed, such as single donor (national authorisation) vs. pooled donor (central authorisation).
>
> (EC DG Enterprise, 2004b)

Although this appeared to be the major organising principle in the first phase, caveats were voiced, especially about relative risks of autologous and allogeneic technologies. The depiction of self-contained autologous applications was predominant, but some stakeholders argued that both types of technology could carry the same level of risk. There was little question that donor-cell based applications would be regulated in an EU-centralised system.

Table 8.2 Is TE special? The original model of a 'third pillar' regulation for tissue-engineered technologies

TISSUES/TISSUE BANKS		TISSUE ENGINEERED PRODUCTS		MEDICINAL PRODUCTS
'Tissues & Cells' Directive		New Regulation		Medicinal Product Regulation
Non-manipulated cells: e.g. cornea, thighbone, blood vessels, skin.	Demarcation based on degree of manipulation	e.g. cultured chondrocytes, engineered skin, cultured myoblasts, unmodified stem cells.	Demarcation based on primary mode of action	e.g. fused cells for cancer vaccines, genetically modified cells. Pharmacologic, immunologic or metabolic modeof action.
		Primary physical or mechanical mode of action.		

Source: Adapted from EuropaBio, 2002 and Chignon, 2003.

Medical device regulation has had wide support from the device industry and is seen as relatively liberal and light-touch compared to medicinal product regulation. Proponents of a 'third pillar' of product regulation, however, regard this regulation as unsuited to the governance of TE technologies. Others believe that existing regulations on cell therapy medicinal products provide a basis for regulation (Kent et al., 2006). The appropriate institutional arrangements continued to be discussed, including the potential role of the EMEA, which is seen negatively by many small companies. New alliances emerged, strengthening relations between different industry sectors. 'Big pharma', biotechnology and medical device companies developed some joint ventures at company level and between trade associations.

During 2004–5, a second major phase of policy negotiation was initiated. The weight of opinion shifted in favour of a distinct regulatory structure located within Europe's existing EMEA. This drew criticism from those stakeholders who preferred to see TE products as '*more devicey*' (as one informant put it) than pharmaceutical. This move paralleled a change of responsibility within EC's DG Enterprise in which tensions in the jurisdictions of medical device and pharmaceutical regulatory regimes were highlighted. The uneasy matching of the organisational with the technological/industrial was further highlighted by apparent territorial disputes within DG Enterprise, between the medicines and medical devices sections. However, the balance of argument now shifted clearly towards the existing pharmaceutical regime.

Pharmaceuticalising devices

By late 2004 a new concept of 'advanced therapies' was emerging into the regulatory arena (EC DG Enterprise and Industry, 2005). The underlying reasons for this about-turn are complex, but in the Commission's rationale it is clear that the prior existence of pharmaceutical regulations and the EMEA loom large, in particular, as noted above, the inclusion of cell therapy medicinal products in an annexe to the Medical Products directive (European Commission, 2003). The logistics, economics and implications for technical expertise of a two-tier system also appear to have been important (EC, 2005).

Via the newly minted concept of advanced therapy, TE was also now being strongly defined by Europe-level officials as part of the biotechnology and pharmaceutical sectors. The debate around a two-tier system geared to national subsidiarity faded away to be replaced by a very strong statement of the need for comprehensive EU-centralised regulation:

> Experience gained in the area of modern biotechnology, where scientific expertise is often limited, highlights the necessity to establish centralised procedures for the authorisation of biotechnology-derived therapeutic products.
>
> (EC DG Enterprise & Industry, 2005)

The issue of risk to human safety was inscribed here as a central organising principle of the forthcoming regulation:

> Traceability from the donor to the patient, long-term patient follow-up and a thorough post-authorisation risk management strategy are crucial aspects to be addressed when evaluating advanced therapies.
>
> (EC DG Enterprise & Industry, 2005: 2)

The framing of the new advanced therapy concept makes a case for the rationale of integrating three types of therapeutic technology as a 'coherent ensemble':

> These three kinds of advanced therapies (gene therapy, somatic cell therapy, and tissue engineering) ... constitute a coherent ensemble:
>
> – Based on complex, highly innovative manufacturing.
> – Pooling of (regulatory and scientific) expertise at Community level is ... essential to ensure a high level of public health protection.
> – Advanced therapy products are usually developed by innovative small and medium-sized enterprises, highly-specialised divisions of larger operators in the Life Science sector (biotechnology, medical devices and pharmaceuticals), hospitals or tissue banks.
>
> (op. cit., 2005)

In fact, EU legislation already existed for cell therapy and gene therapy, so the proposals have a clear emphasis on catering for TE. Advanced Therapy products should be 'intended to be placed on the market in Member States and *either prepared industrially or manufactured by a method involving an industrial process ... Products which are both prepared in full and used in a single hospital, in accordance with a medical prescription for an individual patient, are excluded from the scope of the proposal*' (italics in original). The EC text supplied examples of self-repair (autologous) products which would and would not be covered by the proposed legislation:

> A large operator, operating at global level, developing a product based on autologous cultured chondrocytes, which are manipulated via a well validated and controlled industrial process.
>
> (EC DG Enterprise & Industry, 2005)

And:

> A hospital developing an in-house, non-industrial technology based on autologous cells to repair/regenerate cardiovascular tissue for a given patient. ... neither 'prepared industrially' nor 'manufactured by a method involving an industrial process'.

These examples clearly served a rhetorical purpose. The attempts to distinguish local, patient-specific autologous products from 'industrial' products produced by a standard procedure themselves proved controversial and the issue was debated as 'the hospital exemption'. Even the definition of a 'hospital' was raised, for example by the European Association of Tissue Banks:

> A process of concentration is taking place ... leading to the formation of bigger and major regional and supra-regional tissue banks. The already existing Directive [Tissues and Cells Directive 2004] ... necessitates, in general, a standardised (reproducible) processing. This would appear to overlap with the definitions of 'tissue engineered product' in the proposed regulation.
>
> (EATB, 2005)

In fact there is no legal definition of a hospital in the EU. In the UK, an 'NHS Trust' may comprise several hospitals and other healthcare facilities across several sites, and this issue of hospital networks remains a concern for UK and regulatory officials in some other countries involved with the new regime.

This section has shown that the regulatory ordering of TE, especially illustrated in the policy discourse of new regulation, has framed TE primarily as a special zone of the pharmaceutical regime. 'Advanced therapy' products soon became 'advanced therapy *medicinal* products' in the Commission texts. TE became dubbed as 'unconventional medicine'. However, there remains significant opposition to this move, and significant concern about 'gaps' and ambiguities in the emerging, re-ordered regulatory regime.

Anti-pharmaceuticalisation

A range of national and Europe-level stakeholders, national governments and those directly representing the medical device industry have participated in the regulatory negotiations for tissue-engineered products. A representative of ABHI summarised many of the concerns of the device industry in Europe:

> They [pharmaceutical industry] were dealing with it from a perspective that they had an approach that suited them and which suited their technology – they wanted to fine-tune it ... the device industry said – those are products that are primarily developed by medical device companies ... virtually always have a primary *mechanical* device type of activity ... *don't* extend that [pharmaceutical approach] to things for which it isn't appropriate. And the submissions that we made to the Commission were based ... on the reality of the technology. To take an example, we already implement quality management systems (QMSs), ... if you take the pharmaceutical legislation and apply it to tissue engineering the consequence of that is that a medical device company will now have to have one set of QMSs for most of its products and have a different set of QMSs with a different inspectorate for the rest ... that was not recognised by the ATMP [Advanced Therapy Medicinal Product] regulation ... if you look at the clinical trial regime for drugs it is vastly different to what is done for devices ... The way in which the ATMP was originally drafted would essentially have stifled any device innovation, the compromise which has been reached at the end of the day is not a very happy one ... in the meantime there is the necessity to modify the Medical Device Directives themselves ... there is a grey area where products are going to be misallocated. (For example, a group developing) – substitutes for the liver: what they're seeking to do is to take a matrix which might conceivably be a plastic or more likely to be collagen ... and to grow on that matrix healthy liver cells from the patient's body and then use that as a transplant ... that is *precisely* the kind of technology where the clinicians are up in arms if you say you're going to treat that as a drug.
>
> (Representative of ABHI and Eucomed,
> interview by author, 2007)

Further description of the 'gaps' that the medical device industry might regard as being created by the new advanced therapy regulation have been identified by European trade association Eucomed, in this instance eschewing the EC terminology of 'advanced therapy medicinal product' altogether:

> Human tissue engineered device: Products containing or consisting exclusively of non-viable human cells and/or tissues, which do not contain any viable cells or tissues and which do not act principally by pharmacological, immunological or metabolic action.
>
> (Pirovano, 2007)

Eucomed attempted to influence European parliamentarians in advance of the key Committee of the Environment, Public Health and Consumer Protection (European Parliament) (ENVI) committee and full plenary parliamentary debate of the scope of the new regulation, arguing in the case of combination products:

> a hip joint or a dental implant coated with appropriate cells to facilitate osteointegration could be envisaged ... Where the overall 'therapeutic tool', is clearly a medical device, it would not be appropriate to regulate the whole product under the pharma regime simply because it is coated with human cells. On the other hand, it is obvious that the cellular part needs to be reviewed by analogy according to the ATMP regulation.
>
> (Eucomed, 2007b)

The trade association argued that skills within the Notified Body community (i.e. the EU-wide statutory, delegated, devolved system of device assessment and certification) are specific to the medical devices sector. In relation to proposals in the new regulation for adapting guidelines on good manufacturing practice (GMP) and good clinical practice (GCP) – which are written primarily for pharmaceutical applications, Eucomed asserted that:

> In consideration of the nature of Tissue Engineered Products, we believe that the quality systems and clinical investigation standards, developed for medical devices and other sectors by the International Organisation for Standardisation (ISO) may be more directly relevant.
>
> (Eucomed, 2007b)

The device industry position on advanced therapies has also been supported by the UK government and the devices/medicines regulatory agency:

> We've got a range of points that are important to [government] ministers. ... On the question of the boundaries/overlap between medicines and devices regime, what we would like is to see is clarity ... some of the existing gaps plugged in product regulatory categories ... both medicines and devices regimes available and it be possible to regulate under either regime according to the normal criteria.
>
> (UK regulatory agency official, interview by author, 2006)

This position was confirmed by a government minister:

> in aggregate they [ATMP proposals] do not fully address an existing problem, that some products containing human and animal tissues/cells and used for medicinal purposes fall into gaps between the medicines and medical devices regulatory regimes. We believe that some of these products would continue to be inadequately regulated.
>
> (House of Commons European Scrutiny Committee, 2006: 22)

It is clear, therefore, that the shaping of TE technology as a strand of the pharmaceutical regime is problematic, especially for interests in the Europe-wide medical devices sector. The construction of a TE technological zone in the European institutions cuts uneasily across the boundaries of devices and pharmaceutical regimes. The malleable definition of the material technology, 'the characteristics of the product', are crucial in this regulatory discourse.

Health Technology Assessment of tissue engineered technologies

The UK NICE has reviewed the evidence for ACI twice (NICE, 2000c; 2005). Initially it did not recommend its use for 'routine primary treatment of articular cartilage defects on the knee joint in the NHS', and subsequently it has strengthened this position 'to include all treatment levels':

> all patients receiving ACI should be enrolled in ongoing or new clinical studies; and ... patients should be fully informed of the

uncertainties about the long-term effectiveness and the potential adverse effects of this procedure.

(NICE, 2005a)

The guidance also urged the development of national registries 'to enable the systematic collection of information on long-term outcomes' (NICE, 2005b, press release). Also recommended was further review of alternative treatments, and methodological research into 'the most appropriate way to measure how well the knee functions after surgical and non-surgical treatments' related to a generic measure of health-related quality of life. This expansion of methodological uncertainty is characteristic of much HTA technology appraisal. TE technology has thus become enrolled into the HTA evidentiality movement. The recommendation about national registries is interesting to note, especially in the context of the discussion in this book about the National Joint Registry (NJR) for orthopaedic implants in England and Wales (Chapter 4). It appears that this type of surveillance tool will become more widely deployed in healthcare monitoring and evaluation, possibly at the expense of randomised control trials and other prospective experimental methodologies, whose status as the gold standard of evaluation is being called into question in the case of certain technologies.

The dynamics of tissue engineering governation

The world of medical devices is not a stable one, the world of TE even less so. In this chapter, I have used the case of tissue-engineered technology to highlight the constructed and contingent nature of innovative technologies and a possible newly emerging technological zone. By describing stakeholder contests around the boundary parameters and governance rules of engagement of TE, I have illustrated the interdependence of alternative representations of the material technology and the processes of regulatory regime-building. In order to highlight the constructive nature of the governance processes illustrated in this case study, I introduce the term 'governation'[3]. It is well established that globalisation, the emergence of a 'new political economy' and public sector restructuring within many nation-states internationally is giving rise to new forms and patterns of governance and a 'new public management'. Thus here I suggest that the concept of governation will help in conveying a nuanced understanding of the complex social and discursive processes of regulatory state policymaking that shape a new political economy, of which emerging and evolving biomedical device technologies and technological zones may be part.

In the case of TE as a technological zone, its first decade can be characterised as a struggle, especially by industry and by regulatory policymakers, to create legitimation for a TE identity. As one might expect with a technology that has a limited range of applications in medical practice, accompanied by a wide range of visions and expectations for the future (cf. Brown and Michael, 2003), the governation process has been focused not so much on issues of practical usership and the evaluation of usership outcomes (as with more established device technologies) but more on the definition of the material technology, the structuring of the rules of engagement for the scientific R&D and entrepreneurial arena, the construction of regimes for the sourcing of human tissue materials and debate of appropriate evidential rules for product safety assessment.

I have shown that the aim of policymakers and regulatory regime-builders in the UK has been to promote UK industrial interests in a balanced way. On the European stage this has involved promoting device and pharmaceutical perspectives around definitions of the characteristics of the technology and its benefits and risks. Clinical usership in TE has been constructed more at local level among academic-industrial partnerships, clinical healthcare science evaluations of particular TE applications, representations of clinical experience with patients (for example, wound care ethics) and national HTA evaluations and guidance. In the evidential arena of HTA, the UK healthcare policymaking community, via NICE, has shown itself to be very cautious about TE technology in the form of autologous knee cartilage (ACI) procedure. The gatekeeping rule that patients should only undergo this therapy in the context of a clinical trial is a good example of the uncertainty-containing use of HTA as a boundary organisation between the healthcare state and clinical practice. I have discussed this regulatory positioning of HTA in Chapter 1 as well as elsewhere (Faulkner, 1997). At the same time, NICE, as HTA-based gatekeeper, has urged the extension of prospective monitoring and surveillance data-gathering systems in the case of ACI, thus paralleling the monitoring developments discussed in the other orthopaedic device technology discussed in this book. It may be that the caution here is also influenced by the fact that that this knee cartilage regeneration technology has its main applications in sports medicine, and thus there is a market in private treatment among elite sportspeople.

In terms of evaluation and assessment of TE technologies, pre-marketing product safety approval methodologies have been the major focus of the regulatory regime-building work in the EU, resulting in a proposal for a central EU scientific and technical committee as part of the EMEA (Council of the European Union, 2007). However, 'postmarketing' surveillance was also tackled in the architecture of the Advanced Therapy Medicinal Products regulation. The possibility of databases coordinated and collated cross-nationally and held by an independent monitoring body was discussed in parliamentary and Council of Europe forums, though this level of surveillance did not reach the statute book. Instead, the regulation requires that

> the applicant shall detail, in the marketing authorisation application, the measures envisaged to ensure the follow-up of efficacy of advanced therapy medicinal products and of adverse reactions thereto ... Where there is particular cause for concern, the Commission shall, on the advice of the Agency (EMEA), require ... that a risk management system designed to identify, characterise, prevent or minimise risks ... including an evaluation of the effectiveness of that system, be set up, or that specific post-marketing studies be carried out by the holder of the marketing authorisation and submitted for review to the Agency.
>
> (from Article 15 – Council of the European Union, 2007)

Thus the regulatory requirement is for evidence in the form of specific ad hoc studies, focused on adverse outcomes, rather than a continual surveillance system, and the first line of responsibility is with the manufacturer. This means that for the time being the onus of responsibility will lie also with the regulatory authorities of member states to operate the pharmacovigilance and medical device vigilance reporting systems.

Tissue engineering technology and society

Judged by the evidence of the regulatory regime-building in this case study, the innovation pathways of TE into the healthcare system are unclear, diverse and strewn with obstacles. Stakeholders are struggling to define the parameters of a TE technological zone, and the alignment of such a zone to worlds of clinical practice in a healthcare system is one of many areas of uncertainty and instability. The multiple sources of uncertainty for scientists, industrialists and regulators illustrate the difficulty of locking together the components of a technological pathway in this field. Many TE technologies will follow a pharmaceutical regulatory route for assessment of safety and quality for marketing approval for adoption in the EU, others will be combination products that will be assessed under two regimes, and others may be assessed as medical devices, like the other device technologies discussed in this book.

Theoretical approaches of society/technology studies are applicable to the TE case. I have argued that the processes of regime-building and zone-definition can be characterised as a regulatory ordering (Brown et al., 2006). The trans-national governance of TE is a politico-economic process shaping TE technologies. Governation work results in the shaping of innovation pathways more in some directions than others, for example in foregrounding issues of safety from disease contamination in donor-cell based technologies. The links between a social constructionist perspective and sectoral and distributed 'innovation systems' perspectives are explored somewhat further elsewhere (Faulkner, 2008), as are the links between different framings of risk in this field and their inscription in the new regulatory regime (Faulkner et al., 2008).

While the work of regime-building clearly institutionalises some rules for *participation* in a TE zone in the European healthcare economy, conspicuously absent from this work has been a strong construction of the *usership* of TE technologies in healthcare practice. As colleagues and I have argued elsewhere, the principles of assessment of population-level effectiveness of TE are less prominent in European governation than are the principles of safety assessment, economic viability and competitiveness (Faulkner et al., 2008). The configuring of clinical users is less clear in the architecture of the emerging regime. Likewise, the cautious approach of evidential gatekeeper agencies has been noted, and so here clinical users are shaped as experimentalists rather than routine users. One of the 'problems' with usership here is its diversity across a number of different specialisms. It is notable that it is in the case of cartilage implantation, where the alignment with a medical specialty (orthopaedic surgery) appears much clearer, that the HTA gatekeeping function strongly constrains diffusion of the technology.

TE is becoming framed in industrial and healthcare policymaking communities as part of the new 'regenerative medicine'. Indeed, in the mid-2000s it has become commonplace to refer to a 'regenerative medicine industry'. Such a framing brings TE into the view of social perspectives on issues that in the public sphere are emotive and controversial, especially regarding human embryonic stem cells and inter-species cell manipulations. As we saw in this case study, some end-users may conceive value-based and faith-based concerns about the composition of tissue-engineered technologies. Although this has only been touched on in this chapter, one way in which TE technology configures the (end)-user is as a choice-making consumer and sometimes value-oriented critic of a new form of medicine that acts on the body at a cellular level, potentially invoking a novel set of potentialities for personal identity.

In terms of medicalisation, TE technology is not a 'high-interpretation' technology, in the sense that users may be forced to consider life-changing interpretative decisions on the basis of engagement with it, although in the case of wound care, the issue of knowledge about the composition of TE wound care products may evoke increased engagement of public or patients. Such a move accords with a move towards *bio*medicalisation.

In TE regime-building, the political economy of the healthcare regulatory state works to structure forces shaping a new zone. In this sense, the analysis here goes some way beyond that of a social construction of technology approach, which has been criticised for being oblivious to social structural dynamics (Klein and Kleinman, 2002). These authors:

> define structures as: specific formal and informal, explicit and implicit 'rules of play', which establish distinctive resource distributions, capacities, and incapacities and define specific constraints and opportunities for actors depending on their structural location. Power and its operation are then understood within this structural context.
>
> (Klein and Kleinman, 2002)

The discussion here, in the spirit of this characterisation of structural dynamics, has illustrated interrelationships between industry sectors and government and regulatory agencies at a level of political negotiation of economic and national/supranational interests. In this process, the state's role – here the role of the European regulatory state – has been as analyst of interests, as divided political actor, as classifier of technology and organisation and as orchestrator of rules of engagement ('rules of play' above) for a pan-European technological zone. In this process it is impossible to ignore the close proximity of regulators and industrial representatives, in spite of structural and cultural divisions between the different interested industry sectors. Thus, in the UK, the state's role combines a strong bi-sectoral industry advocacy with healthcare system gatekeeping via HTA intermediary organisations.

TE technologies in contemporary healthcare, in summary, have low levels of credibility, healthcare usership and societal acceptance. The widely known issues of ethics associated with some aspects of the field have been separated from the politico-economic regulatory regime building (.Faulkner et al., 2006). TE has avoided controversy related to those technologies already in clinical practice. The salience of the materiality of the technology in regulatory political discourse suggests that the theoretical approaches of Actor-Network Theory (ANT) and 'technology-in-practice' are applicable in this case (cf. Timmermans and Berg, 2003a). These overlapping approaches to understanding the conundrums of society/technology highlight the dynamic mutual constitution of social, institutional and material actors in this field.

9
Devising Healthcare and Society

The origin of the HTA movement in the UK can be traced to a pivotal conference early in the 1990s that announced the dangers to society of a 'Tidal Wave' of new medical technologies (Advisory Group on HTA, ca. 1992). The image – a determinist vision, no doubt – of a tsunami of technological innovation, to which health policymakers, scientists and evaluators, regulators and the wider society had to respond, was a powerful one. There was much concern, voiced in forums such as the *British Medical Journal* and shared widely across the advanced industrialised nations, of the dangers of 'unevaluated' technologies, and of the allegedly high proportions of technologies already diffused and routinised in the healthcare system for which evidence of effectiveness and cost-effectiveness was non-existent. Since then, the explosion in healthcare evidentiality has started to redress this situation, but it also, paradoxically, continues to illuminate the extent of ignorance and lack of research-based knowledge of the performance of medical technologies. As a sometime practitioner of HTA myself, I have sought to treat evidentiality, from a sociological viewpoint, not as the sole means of addressing the problems of technological healthcare, but as one of several dynamic forces at the entry-points, gatekeeping spaces and innovation pathways between medical technology innovation and the healthcare system. To do this it has been necessary to develop some understanding of the world of medical devices and the medical devices industrial sector, which have been shown to be part and parcel of the healthcare state. I have aimed to explore the shaping of medical technology and the medical-technological shaping of society, and the parts played by science and governance in these relations. I have drawn on, illustrated and analysed evidence of general trends, for example the incrementalist approach to innovation in the medical device industry, and of specific device technologies, to show that patterns of science and governance differ significantly between types of device, and that comparison of such patterns will yield a better understanding of the complex dynamics of innovation pathways into healthcare.

The book, therefore, engages with a number of recent programmes for the sociological study of medical technology and governance. For example, understanding of the core dynamics of the contemporary world of medicine, it has been recommended, now requires a combination of attention to political economy and the medical sociologist's more traditional qualitative analysis of the social meanings of medicine (Conrad, 2005). Likewise, studies in sociology 'have not fully examined the complexity of how (technology) governance is achieved' (Fox et al., 2007).

The book offers case studies in the forces shaping public experience of medical device technologies through healthcare systems, and thus the shaping of the consumption of healthcare risks and benefits. This in turn reflexively re-shapes the parameters of the methodologies for the production of healthcare science and evidence. The construction of public and policy concerns about safety, efficacy and effectiveness, and the societal acceptability of each considered device technology differs. This final discussion draws together the strands that have been laid out in the case study chapters. Firstly, I compare and discuss the pathways of device innovation in the healthcare system and governance processes interacting with them. I explore the variation in the scientific evidentiality and the configuring of social-organisational relations of governance. And secondly, I pick up the theoretical threads from the introductory parts of the book, and the concluding sections of the case study chapters, to develop theoretical understanding of the societal dynamics of contemporary health technology innovation and governance. This discussion draws especially on the various concepts and perspectives which I introduced earlier as constituting the conundrum of technology/society – social shaping, co-construction, usership, domestication, the configurability and obduracy of material technology, medicalisation and industry-healthcare-state relations. I also bring forward a discussion of a theme in the relationship of technology and society that has been latent in my portrayal of the world of medical devices and the particular device technologies that I have presented as case studies, namely the varying ways that discourses of '*risk*' have been produced and mobilised.

Specific devices, big trends

The device technologies that I have studied are to some extent representative of 'big trends' in contemporary healthcare and society. They have significance as exemplars of many of the major trends that characterise contemporary medicine and healthcare in the advanced industrial societies. Notable trends exemplified here include the intensification of the healthcare workplace, development of regenerative medical paradigms, increasing implantability and biocompatibility of technology, health *service* risk amplification and institutionalisation, evidentiality – new forms of scientific evidence and evaluation, corporatisation/privatisation in public welfare systems, citizen-patient empowerment movements, blame-free and participative organisational culture, technological interconnectivity and informaticisation, distributedness of data and material of the human body (cf. Brown & Webster, 2004, especially on the last two trends). Thus the devices that I have examined are part of the world of medical devices but also constitute challenges to the always-renegotiable boundaries of that world. However, a key outcome of my analysis is that these trends are not uniform, generic or evenly distributed across all of healthcare – there are technology-specific and zone-specific innovation pathways.

Five devices – innovation-governance patterns compared

The five case studies provide contrasting and overlapping pictures (or, better, videos) of patterns of material technology, stakeholder interest, usership, evidentiality and governance involved in their innovation and diffusion in the healthcare system. These are summarised in Table 9.1. Clearly, a first conclusion to be drawn is that few of the innovation 'pathways' that technology producers or healthcare professionals or healthcare commissioners or patient groups might like to envisage are clear, straightforward or unobstructed. The respective patterns of powers of stakeholders and discourses in the material technology, usership, evidence and governance vary strikingly between devices. Many conflicting tensions between trends and stakeholders have been illustrated in each case. Here, I note the most conspicuous features of each device technology in the development of its configuration of innovation-shaping dynamics. Following the structure of the case study chapters, I first highlight the key points related to innovation pathways, evidentiality (pointing out the forms of evidence that have become most salient for the innovation pathway and governance process) and governance.

Artificial hips

The case study shows a device that has been highly successful clinically, commercially and for patients. US-dominated multinational commercial interests continuously produce technological innovation in design and materials. The design cannot be said to be stabilised, although there are some established features that apply for most clinical populations. Producers seek to extend the technology to both younger and older patient groups. Thus there are now fewer companies, producing a wider variety of prostheses. The designs show a trend toward 'hip systems' giving surgeons a range of sizes, materials and so on. Close relations between surgeons and the orthopaedic device industry were evident. In the early 1990s, in the UK, the major governance issue was cost-effectiveness related to the proliferation of models, and it was one of the first technologies to be assessed with the developing systematic review methods of HTA. This uncovered the array of different prostheses diffused into the healthcare system and geographical variations in practice, and elite surgeons embracing EBM began to warn about 'designer hips'. Also highlighted was the lack of methodologically robust evaluation – 'evidence' – of alternative hip designs. Towards the end of the 1990s and into this century, hip prostheses and orthopaedic practices attracted a very high level of government and regulatory attention, and self-scrutiny by the orthopaedic profession also grew. This resulted in a degree of self-regulation through professional guidelines, and the HTA strand of regulatory evidentiality resulted in guidance for the NHS produced by the then NICE, which drew on the '10-year rule' – no more than 10 per cent failure rate at 10 years' lifetime of prosthesis – already negotiated between the profession and the national regulatory agency (the then MDA, under the EU medical device system). However, the subsequent '3-year rule' permits new models to be introduced on the basis of relatively short follow-up data. The incident of the apparent, though disputed, failure of the *Capital* hip system led to heightened professional and political concern, and calls for surveillance through a 'registry' system increased. Apparently minor design variants on a gold standard technology could be the cause of major clinical problems. Upward reclassification of the risk status of the prosthesis under the EU regulatory regime increased the level of requirement for *clinical* evidence for market approval of 'new' devices. Latterly, governance via NICE guidance in the UK was supplemented by a move towards control at the point of national and regional procurement – the establishment of an orthopaedic data evaluation panel to collect early data from manufacturers on new designs of prosthesis. A National Joint Registry (NJR) has been established.

Thus over 15 years the orthopaedic device industry subsector's incrementalist approach to innovation, resulting in diversification of designs, fixation methods and materials, became associated with a high degree of evidential uncertainty produced through the emerging healthcare sciences and professional introspection. The healthcare sciences were enrolled into governance activity, which then itself diversified in an attempt to regulate the continued expansion of hip prosthesis technologies. In spite of the increasing level of governance activity, especially through surveillance and data collection, from a public health perspective the gatekeeping effect to date appears weak (van der Meulen, 2005). The reversibility of the main parameters of this innovation pathway is low, though some newer variants (such as 'porous-coating') are at the centre of evidential contests between stakeholders.

The PSA test

The use of this blood test technology, a pre-diagnostic aid, is widely diffused throughout cancer-related healthcare services, and it is also available via self-testing kits. Like artificial hips, it attracted the attention of the early development of HTA in the UK, as elsewhere. Subsequently, it has become, in financial terms, of the highest priority in the UK's HTA programme. In this case, however, the original policy 'problem' was the issue of the possible introduction of mass screening for prostate cancer. The initial national-level guidance was shaped through a national NHS HTA review organisation. The framing of state requirements for new evidence about PSA testing was controversial in terms of both methodology and ethics, which were closely entangled. Patients and potential patients have been shown to have highly divergent views about the value and personal significance of the test associated with the interpretation of its results. It has highlighted stakeholder conflict between proponents (e.g. cancer charities and some urological surgeons) and opponents (public health communities, official government). The extreme scientific evidential uncertainty surrounding usership of the technology and prostate cancer treatment had been diffused to citizens both via mega-scale population HTA studies and by government 'risk management' policy with which it is closely allied. Both science and governance have constructed a policy of 'informing' men of the uncertainties, and doing so in a form of counselling. Thus citizens have been enrolled into a mode of governance which promotes a sharing of the risks associated with deployment of the test. Medical diagnostics science and industry are developing variants of the basic technology, but while these may perform better as predictive tools, the interpretative uncertainty remains. Governance attempts to control the diffusion of PSA testing have been relatively unsuccessful, *de facto* screening having 'crept in by the back door' at an increasing rate. The commitment of the surgical profession to radical treatments is one factor in this and healthcare professionals' practice of defensive medicine another (advising the test as a precaution in case of missing a cancer diagnosis). Thus the innovation pathway into healthcare of PSA technology is characterised by a plateau-like state, containing conflicting professional and public interests, associated with the uncertainty maintained by HTA science and a social legitimation of this through a strategic diffusion of 'risk' to citizens.

Infusion pumps

This device technology is notable for the part played by concepts of error and scientific investigation of usership and failure in its governance. The problems identified with infusion pumps revolve around proliferation of models of the device and complexity of operating it by users, primarily nurses. The user interface is central to the device governance that has been developed. An 'evaluation gap' in the regulatory regimes was highlighted. More than the other devices discussed here, the problems of this device have been framed in terms of 'safety' though this has been formulated in different frames by different regulatory-evidential agency constituencies. Unlike artificial hips and the PSA test, the healthcare science of HTA has not (yet) been prominent in the innovation pathway of the technology. Most obviously, the issues of infusion pumps have been framed by the UK's unique National Patient Safety Agency (NPSA), and like artificial hips there has recently been a move to construct governance at the point of procurement, in an attempt at standardisation. There is evidence of clashing interpretations of the definition of regulatory jurisdictions between the device approval agency working under the EU MDD and the patient safety agency. Technologically, the innovation pathway is towards increasing incorporation of software functions and electronic communication and database features. These 'smart' devices aim to introduce increased in-built safety features, but the current evaluations raise uncertainty about the usability and effectiveness of these innovations in the work organisation. The innovation pathway in the healthcare system can be characterised as one of reliance upon this technology, accompanied by multifaceted governance as damage or risk minimisation. The case study shows a move in regulatory governance towards a construction of events of performance failure as an attribute of organisational systems of healthcare.

Coagulometer

This case study is the only one in this book where a technology for home-based healthcare is the primary focus. It is conspicuous also because the device itself is not available in the UK through the NHS – it can be purchased in the commercial marketplace. Nevertheless, the *use* of this self-monitoring device has been negotiated as part of the public healthcare system. It thus straddles the boundary between the private marketplace and public care. Associated with these features of the innovation in self-monitoring anticoagulation therapy, the device has become part of the activities of patient advocacy and support groups. A small number of clinical champions, allied with diagnostics industry, promote the device in the UK. The market for a self-monitoring device is dominated worldwide by a single manufacturer, although others show signs of entering. Although the size of the potential usership is large, the diffusion of the device to date is modest. The focus of evidential governance has been on uncoordinated studies of clinical effectiveness and to some extent cost-effectiveness. These show that self-monitoring has as good or better effectiveness and safety as hospital-based haematology clinics. There are contested clinical concerns about risks related to 'excessive' rates of monitoring. Latterly, UK HTA systematic review methods have begun to move towards a coordinated assemblage of evidence in a national and international (Cochrane Collaboration) scientific framework. Governance concerns about the use of the device focus around the healthcare/homecare boundary and the implications for reconfiguration of accountabilities, the competence of users and technological quality control versus performance standards. The case study identified a lack of research evidence about users' experience of the device and how the interpretation of its monitoring data interacts with people's understanding of personal metabolism and other variable embodied experience. The innovation pathway is open to shaping by governmental forces as demonstrated by the relatively high rate of diffusion in Germany under the impetus of state-supported programmes and conducive legislation. Exploration of technological development of the device is focused on ICT communication features and capability of linking to electronic patient records. The UK state remains an arm's length participant in the governance of the technology – the state regulatory agencies that feature in the other case studies in this book are not prominent as gatekeepers to the healthcare system. Clinical and healthcare constituencies are cautious for evidential and resourcing reasons, though there are signs that a coordinated national healthcare R&D mandated large-scale clinical trial will be constructed, which would undoubtedly increase the pressure for wider adoption of the technology.

Tissue-engineered technologies

This case study differed from the others in a number of ways. Firstly, the case study does not deal with a single type of device (leaving aside for the moment the issue of diversification, hybridisation and connectivity of 'single' device types). Secondly, the focus was on Europe-level governation processes, rather than UK processes. Thirdly, it is more concerned with the contested processes of constructing a new regulatory regime than it is with the institutional configuring of agencies and actors in the governation of healthcare system-specific technological innovation.

TE is being positioned contentiously across the boundaries of the politico-economic identities of medical devices on the one hand, and pharmaceuticals on the other. As a (possibly) emerging technology and scientific-industrial zone, the governation process of TE has been focused not so much on issues of practical usership and the evaluation of usership outcomes (as with more established device technologies such as artificial hips and infusion pumps), but on the definition of the material technology, the structuring of the rules of engagement for the scientific and entrepreneurial participants, the construction of regimes for the sourcing of human tissue and appropriate evidential rules for product safety assessment. I illustrated the deep divide between stakeholders in medical device and pharmaceutical sectors and how this revolved around constructions of the material technology of TE itself. In terms of evidentiality, premarketing product safety approval methodologies have been the major focus of the regulatory regime-building work in the EU, though the Europe-level regime and the UK HTA-based regime both have promoted surveillance-based methods of monitoring of clinical patient outcomes.

Overall, the case studies indicate evidence of a tendency for increased *coordination* of evidence-related forms of governance. This is seen especially in the use of the HTA systematic review method to amalgamate clinical data from diverse sources and in movements to establish wide-ranging data reporting, monitoring and surveillance systems. Standardisation through 'evidence-based' purchasing and procurement policy is a notable feature of governance activity in the case of the electromedical equipment example (infusion pumps) and the well-established implantable device (artificial hips). There is a notable diversification of governance agencies becoming involved in these technologies.

Table 9.1 Five devices – innovation-governance patterns compared

Technology Issues	Innovation pathway characteristics	Usership	Advocacy	Salient science/ evidence	Governance configuration
Artificial hips proliferation, cost/effectiveness, safety	Widespread, many incremental variants and hybridisation, regional practices	Orthopaedic surgeons, Patients (end-user)	Industry, Surgeons	HTA special govt. inquiries, incident investigation, practice patterns	EU Directive NICE guidance Professional Surveillance-Registry Procurement
PSA test interpretive uncertainty, diffusion, risk	Ubiquitous, development of some variants	Urological surgeons, Oncologists, General practitioners, Citizens/patients	Cancer charities Some clinicians Some patients Industry	HTA and HSR, Mega-trials, practice patterns	Government risk management, National Professional 'market' of citizen choice
Infusion pumps proliferation, complexity, safety, work organisation	Ubiquitous, software & comms. links, user interface and workplace developments	Nurses, pharmacists, clinical engineers, Patients (end-user)	Industry, Healthcare system	Adverse incident reporting, monitoring systems, device evaluation, usership science	EU Directive Diverse regulators Surveillance reporting/ monitoring, Training & risk management, Procurement

Coagulometer safety, cost/effectiveness, healthcare/society interfaces	Small-scale, growing, poss. communication technology, ambiguous public service (NHS) status	Citizens/patients as purchaser/consumer – linked to healthcare, Industry professional	Patients, patient groups, Industry, Some clinicians	Uncoordinated clinical studies, growing national HTA, Technical device evaluation	Market Local professional
Tissue-engineering safety, economics, ethics	Very small-scale, specialised clinical application Emerging or faltering or diversifying? Developments under trial	specialist health professional Patients (burns victims, athletes, chronic ulcer) future coronary, organ failure, others	lobbyists – EU Parliament, Industry, DTI, biotech sciences, 'Europe' National healthcare	Clinical – trials, surveillance, innovative science, social/ethics	EU Regulation MHRA – voluntary guidance for industry; NICE

In contrast, in the cases of the uptake of the coagulometer and the PSA test, both technologies where the end-user, as citizen or as patient, and the marketplace of informed patient choice are to the fore, the governance regimes have emphasised carefully controlled innovation into the healthcare system, connected to elaborate programmes of selective training and information-provision in the one case and generalised diffusion of risk information in the other. In the case of PSA, the central government in the UK has taken an active role, while with the coagulometer, localised, uncoordinated clinical champions and patient advocate groups have been the innovating actors, often in alliance with the leading device manufacturer. This pattern has been matched by small-scale clinical studies with the coagulometer and large-scale national HTA mega-trials around the PSA test. Interestingly, the sequential development of HTA science has moved from systematic review to large-scale trial in the case of PSA, and from trials *to* systematic review in the case of the coagulometer. There may be a more widespread cyclic phenomenon at work here. Finally, in the analysis of TE technology, the conflictual boundary between the zone of a pharmaceuticalised definition of TE and the sector of medical devices was highlighted.

I now move on to consider medical devices in terms of the conundrum of society/technology, drawing on the accounts that I have set out in the case study chapters. I consider comparisons between the technologies and common threads in terms of a number of the themes introduced in the early chapters of the book. This concluding discussion, therefore, covers technological connectivity and convergence, the political economy of the technological healthcare state, the construction and practices of risk, medicalisation and the varieties of usership of medical devices, related to issues of the configurability of technology.

Medical device technology and society

Technological systems – diversification and connection

One of the big trends in technological healthcare is the growing interdependence of technologies, their hybridisation and diversification through small design and material variants and their increasing incorporation of biotechnology and ICT linkage. All five device technologies examined in this book exemplify this in one way or another. In the case of artificial hips, where 'me-too' technologies have proliferated, the tension between diversification and convergence has been described in detail elsewhere (Neary, 2007). At this point it is useful to return to the notion of technological system associated with the work of Hughes

(1983), which I introduced in Chapter 1. The key notion here is that its innovation is seen as the result largely of small, developing modifications, rather than breakthrough moments. The case studies in this book have furnished a number of examples of this, some where the development has originated primarily with designers and developers, and some where users such as surgeons or nurses have been closely involved. In the case of infusion pumps, we saw detailed evidence of interaction between manufacturer and the general usership following reporting of device failures. Thus the current search among healthcare policy networks for the next 'disruptive' technology (Christensen, 2000) is a search for the exceptional.

Convergence of technologies is an area of interest in industrial policy. For example, in the UK advanced wound management and orthopaedic technologies are currently seen as one interface where new product innovation from TE is becoming linked to the orthopaedic device subsector (DTI, 2005). Clearly, the 'engineering' involved here is of the heterogeneous kind – governments involve themselves in creating the conditions in which interdisciplinary scientific networks might be steered towards convergent technology development. Thus the agencies of the regulatory state themselves can be characterised as heterogeneous engineers at the 'macro' level of the political economy, in the same way that professional engineers or surgeons are at the level of inter-organisational and interdisciplinary interactions. The move towards regenerative medicine, as shown in the accounts of TE and artificial hips in this book, is taking place at the uneasy and contested intersection between the pharmaceutical and medical device industrial sectors: drives toward technological connectivity, therefore, may be obstructed and re-routed by problems of alignment with existing sectoral organisation and regulatory and evidential regimes.

The account in this book of infusion pumps (and coagulometers to a lesser extent) provided evidence of the incorporation of informatics features into the device. For infusion pumps, this includes both programmability of the device itself and electronic connectivity with hospital-based drug management databases and rules and networking of multiple pumps on a site. As I will explore below, many of these innovations introduced by developers have been made in response to a growing awareness of risks associated with the devices and their use in hospital workplaces. The growing interdependence of medical devices and organisational informatics systems may be leading to particular forms of 'lock-in' between hybrid technologies such as this. Thus such developments create technological systems where one technology shapes another and they become interdependent. Of course, this does not amount to a form of technological determinism, as even this brief discussion has indicated – a range of social, economic and political actors are involved in constructing and negotiating the direction that such systems might take. It is clear that some technologies have characteristics that are in principle conducive to adaptive learning in the organisation of healthcare. More 'discrete' technologies will become stabilised in healthcare and medical practice, if at all, by other means. I return to this issue of configurability and discreteness of medical device technology below.

Political economy, healthcare state and technological knowledge

The pre-eminence of the medical profession in steering the adoption of new device technologies has been challenged for some time, in historical, social and economic trends that have been well documented (Gabe et al., 1994; Kelleher et al., 2006). The contemporary global world of medical devices is constituted by an array of more or less powerful actors, such as industry, capital, material technology, science, engineering, markets, healthcare systems and providers, healthcare workers, policymakers, regulators, governments, clinical scientists and end-users and patients. In this book I have used Moran's (1999) terminology of the healthcare state to indicate the close interpenetration of governance, the national healthcare system and the medical devices/healthcare products industries. Most, though not all, of the device technologies which I have studied here are supported by strong commercial development and promotion. I have referred in Chapter 2 to new concepts of medicalisation that embrace notions of corporate medicine (Conrad, 2005) and the techno-science of biomedicine (Clarke et al., 2003). Evidence in this book of such an institutionalising nexus of interests comes from TE in the close relationship of industry representatives and regulatory policymakers in the building of a new regulatory regime, from artificial hips in the integration of device manufacturers in the orthopaedic registry surveillance system and in the 'evidence-based' national NHS procurement agency, and from infusion pumps in the industry's technological innovations framed in line with safety-focused governance developments. However, it is important to note that the 'nexus' is neither ubiquitous nor even across all types of healthcare technology. Here it is useful to recall the analysis of Blume (1992), which I noted in Chapter 2, in his study of the development of diagnostic imaging technologies – evidence that neither technological determinism nor capitalist industrial domination provided accurate accounts, and that negotiated integration of medical and industrial interests were at the root of the innovation process.

Crucial to the industrial economy of healthcare are highly politicised issues of privatisation of public services. Here I do not explore the social, political and ethical critiques of privatisation, nor evidence of its extent in the UK or elsewhere. However, the device technologies that I have described provide examples of linkage between the device industry and device usership that require interpretation. Thus in the cases of infusion pumps, coagulometers and artificial hips, there is evidence that particular multinational companies have created device-specific or family-of-devices-specific networks of relationships with users – patients, patient advocacy groups, surgeons and other clinicians, nurses, hospital management and procurement agencies. For example, particular models of artificial hips require particular equipment for the surgery and the company provides subsidised training to surgeons in that technology; infusion pump manufacturers develop programming and ICT functions in their pump technology that 'requires' dedicated training and is associated with the development of linked infusion 'safety systems' that are proprietary to the developers. Thus in these instances, it is clear that an interdependence is created that has the marks of territorial market-building activity. Surgical and medication system–related expertise is codified into such sociotechnological systems; it is privatised in the sense that access to that expertise is part of a contract between commercial supplier and the institutional device-user.

Regulation, governance and governation

The movement from government towards forms of governance associated with the neoliberal state and deregulation underlies much of the governance activity portrayed in this book. It is axiomatic that regulatory regime-building around technology constitutes a 'fluid governance jigsaw' (Brown et al., 2006) and that technology governance is 'forever breaking down and being reinvented to address societal changes' (Fox et al., 2007). In my account of the technological zone of TE, I introduced the term 'governation' to indicate the constructive, inventive action of stakeholders in the European regulatory state in shaping the boundaries and rules of engagement for that piece of the evolving jigsaw puzzle of technological healthcare. The case studies in this book have illustrated the varying patchworks of regulatory activity in the distributed governance of the healthcare state. In this short section I interpret the actors and agencies of governation, further using some of the case study evidence.

The case studies provided examples of the incorporation of information and communication technology into the hardware of medical devices. Chapter 3 noted the importance of classification in defining an industrial sector or zone, and its importance in processes of regulatory regime-building, and in issues of alignment between technology producer and healthcare users. It is thus useful to note that recent EU-level review of the Medical Device Directives (MDDs) has resulted *inter alia* in the inclusion of computer software in the regulatory boundaries of medical devices. Thus the evolving governance process re-creates the boundaries of the regulatory regimes, regimes for assessment of safety and efficacy are extended, and a perhaps uneasy tension is defined between the world of medical devices and the world of software development. Software becomes a medical device through a governance process.

A similar analysis can be made in the case of the other devices. Interactive governance processes shape the latest technology development issue for infusion pumps as one of 'safety systems'. For the PSA test it produces the informed citizen, uncertain and counselled, at the borders of healthcare and society; for the coagulometer, where the commercial marketplace together with local healthcare professional communities are the main 'regulator', the lack of state governation shapes an innovation space where local gatekeeping and industry interactions are key.

Apart from enabling and shaping technology innovation, regulation is often assumed to be undertaken in order to engender 'public trust'. However, it may be that the advance of regulatory evidentiality has complex effects in this regard. 'Regulation by information' (Majone, 1997) is important in the regulatory state, as the case studies in this book testify, and it appears that there is a paradox of increasing the societal credibility of governance arrangements, which at the same time produces greater exposure to evidential uncertainties among citizens, patients and other technology users. Public trust *may* be engendered both by the regulatory diffusion of uncertainty, as in the PSA test, or by the containment of uncertainty, as with infusion pumps and artificial hips. The active agents of governation shape society's access to and experience of these differing technologies in differentiated processes of trust-building and social legitimation.

Discourses and practices of risk

I have deliberately avoided discussing 'risk' as a primary concept in the case studies or introductory parts of this book. It is an over-used and overly broad term in sociological studies of medicine and health (where are the sociological analyses of benefit?), and it is easy for it to become enmeshed in grand theoretical analysis of the hypothesised 'risk society' and the like. However, of course, the hazards of healthcare and its technologies are important (to health, and politically and analytically), and the construction of *hazards as* risks in regulatory and health policy discourse is a crucial aspect of the governance of health technology innovation. As colleagues and I have discussed elsewhere, the societal framing of technology-related risks increasingly has become closely related to, but not necessarily matching or interlocked with, modes of governance in 'risk regulation' regimes (Faulkner et al., 2008). It is important to understand how risk is being discursively framed and constructed, and institutionalised and acted upon.

In this book, a summary of the risk discourses across the five technologies shows evidence of risk defined in terms of many different dimensions: human physical safety, human or system error, scientific evidential uncertainty, citizen decision-making uncertainty, 'technical' performance (itself constituted in various dimensions), healthcare system cost, system-level clinical effectiveness, social values and ethics. Typically, several different framings of risk have been produced around the same device by different stakeholders and participants. It appears that this phenomenon is not a simple matter of different 'types' of technology evoking different types of socially shaped risk by some direct process of translation, though this is a factor: each device shows a variable pattern of social and technological 'shaping'. Why, for example, has a discourse of 'safety' become dominant in the case of infusion pumps, but not in the case of artificial hips? Why has a discourse framed in the terminology of 'risk' itself – and risk management – become particularly prominent in the political governance of PSA testing?

In the case of the infusion pump, contributing factors have been the link to the broader policy discourse of medication errors and the occasional exposure of news of fatalities in the public sphere. Here, society in the form of healthcare regulatory governance and in the form of 'social concern' mediated and amplified by government and the broadcast media, have elevated risk issues in the form of 'patient safety' issues. The link to the high safety–risk assessment and practices of the aviation industry has been particularly salient in the move towards a patient safety culture in which risk is formulated as primarily a property of organisational systems that may lead to incidents, and which require standardisation not only of the user interface of the device, but what might be termed the workplace interface – in which proliferation of devices is a problem for users. In contrast, the risks of artificial hips were framed primarily in terms of a healthcare evaluation agenda of effectiveness and cost-effectiveness, constructed through application of the healthcare sciences to issues of a proliferation of 'untested' models. The 'Capital' hip system incident erupted into this arena, drawing a discourse of safety that was not prominent otherwise (though it was not associated with fatalities). The extreme governation activity around this incident made the risk discourse more complex by giving added emphasis to human safety concerns, and the EU, influenced partly by UK regulatory impetus, upgraded the safety risk classification of hip prostheses in the EU system. Although the aim was to identify the 'root cause' of the apparent device failure, the regulatory investigation in fact concluded with a recommendation about 'the system', a similar formulation of risk to that seen with infusion pumps. In the case of the PSA test, the prevailing risk assessment and governance discourse has not been one of safety. My account of it showed that uppermost was a discourse of 'risk' of prostate cancer and of risk of knowledge or uncertainty for patients/citizens associated with the imprecise quasi-diagnostic results produced by the technology. The case study showed the massive variation in men's evaluations of the value and significance of the technology. Thus in this case the risk discourse was strongly associated with the broader discourse in population health policy about the benefits and disbenefits of disease screening programmes, a contested governance arena that also includes, for example, mammography.

Thus, the relationship between framings of risk and device technologies is not only artefactually shaped but is also shaped by variable social forces such as scientific risk assessment criteria, linkage to risk discourse in domains other than healthcare and the activity of regulatory political actors.

Technological medicalisation

Medicalisation remains a key concept in considering effects and interactions between technologised medicine and society, as I noted in Chapter 2. In terms of the conundrum of society/technology, medicalisation is a usefully hybrid concept. It highlights the medical sector as an arena in which technology and society meet; it has the flexibility to refer to social and to technological forces in variable combinations. It is thus conducive to various forms of co-construction that can be discerned in the dynamics of medicine, healthcare, state and social process.

The book has conceptualised medicine primarily in terms of healthcare system and industry as co-producers of technological healthcare.

Usership has been conceptualised as a sometimes active consumption of device technologies, inside the healthcare system by patients and health professionals, and outside it by citizens. The malleability of these twin statuses is one of the sources of ambivalence in the social experience of interaction with medical devices. The outdated concept of medicalisation as a unidirectional process in which the medical profession and its knowledge, expertise, language and institutions encroached upon society is now recognised as unhelpful. The case studies in this book, by contrast, provide evidence of the 'complex, ambiguous and contested' (Ballard and Elston, 2005) nature of contemporary medicalisation and demedicalisation. Medical device technology thus deserves attention as one strand of contemporary medicalisation processes. As Conrad (2005) noted, this manifests itself both at the level of the political economy and the level of more direct interaction between medical provision and members of society, the two main lines of analysis that I have followed in this book. The interpenetration of the regulatory state and the healthcare system changes the nature of medicalisation, as does the technologisation of medical and healthcare practice.

One form of technological medicalisation is the scientific industry-based extension of technological healthcare to medical conditions not previously catered for and to patient groups not previously configured as recipients for existing forms of medical technology. This is illustrated in this book by the cases of tissue engineering (TE) and of artificial hips, the former shown in the market-building activity of the regulatory classification of an emerging technological zone, and the latter in the technology-based extension of hip replacement to more elderly and more youthful citizens.

Ambivalent medicalisation is represented, for example, by the home-based coagulometer. The case study showed that, on the one hand, the developers and distributors of the device, linked with and supported by patient advocacy groups, inscribe a blueprint of enhancement of personal autonomy, empowerment and independence in their vision of the device, while on the other hand (although empirical research is lacking here), the continual availability of this hand-held monitoring device to people with potentially life-threatening conditions and sensitive drug therapy might represent a psychological burden – the constant presence of a connection to disease and healthcare professionals, which might be experienced as an ever-present imperative to (over-)monitor one's blood-thinning therapy. Demedicalisation and medicalisation are both present here. It should not be assumed that 'home-based' means non-medicalised. A similar ambivalence is evident in the case of the PSA test. Here, the case study showed that the technology was associated with a healthcare evidentiality and a government-promoted diffusion of uncertainty about the value of the test, related to its flexible interpretability. Thus medicalisation here, in a reversal of the traditional notion of the encroachment of medical authority, signals a diffusion of medical ignorance in which citizens are presented with the existential dilemma of whether, in essence, to embrace or oppose medicalisation.

The rise of a safety culture is said to be characteristic of many sectors of late modern society. I discussed in the previous section the varieties of discourses of risk related to medical devices, and the specificity of safety as one formulation of risk in regulatory governance activity. Thus one aspect of medicalisation associated with infusion pump technology, especially given the very large numbers of health service workers using them, is a practical engagement with the social trend of safety culture. As I noted in the case study chapter, there is a paradoxical medicalisation associated with this technology. On the one hand, contemporary pump technology enables more complex and tailored regimes of medication, while on the other the development of interconnected proprietary ICT-based safety systems represents a form of privatisation of expertise in healthcare practice that indicates the extension of corporate medicine. Thus the development of such technologies amounts to a reconfiguring of the machinery of medicalisation. The question of whether the development of safety systems may compromise safe operations (Perrow, 1999) in the case of the emerging infusion pump information and communication systems, should be the subject of empirical investigation in the healthcare and social sciences.

Technological medicalisation, therefore, is complex in its device-related forms. The social meanings of technological healthcare are not straightforward, and society through evidential assessments, through information-gathering and through regulatory regimes seeks to shape the interface between civil society and the technological healthcare system and its medical devices. Individual citizens, in the case of some technologies, construct the meanings of medical devices with similar ambivalence.

Configurability, interpretability, usership and citizenship

The case study of TE in this book showed how the 'deviceness' of medical devices, and the pharmaceutical identity of tissue engineered technologies, are defined by boundary-making governation activity that depended upon the malleability of the material technology of TE, what the scholars in the Social Construction of Technology tradition would have called its 'interpretative flexibility'. Thus the classificatory boundaries of deviceness, like those of other groupings of technology such as 'cell therapy' or 'xenotransplantation' or 'blood', are negotiable. This book has given many examples of the social, political and economic actors and agencies that involve themselves in attempting to shape and promote particular versions of what a technology is, and how its social usership should be understood and influenced. Yet medical device technologies, to greater or lesser extents, and in different ways, appear constructed with characteristics that either resist or facilitate re-invention and re-interpretation. In this final discussion, therefore, I return to the conundrum of society/technology to examine the differential construction of relationships between types of (socio)technology and (techno)social actors.

Types of technology, types of social actor, and usership

In Chapter 2, I discussed different concepts that have been developed for classifying technology. In the case studies, I have drawn attention at some points to the notion that some technologies appear more 'obdurate' than others, and that some appear more open to the intervention of their users. Some appear to be *more* interpretatively flexible, or open to domestication, at particular points, than others. I discussed also the theoretical analysis of what I have called usership, calling into question the 'artificial' design-use interface. The cases of the PSA test and the coagulometer, in particular, highlighted the question of whether their 'users' could justifiably be conceptualised as such, or whether a broader concept of social actor or citizenship was more appropriate. Citizens using or confronted with these technologies occupied ambivalent statuses, moving between patient and citizen, between marketplace consumer and healthcare recipient, between device trainee and device-use expert, between the informed choice-maker and the counselled, collaborative care-participant. Structuring the dynamics of these identities was the political and industrial economy of the healthcare state and stakeholder governation processes that I have illustrated.

The innovation pathway of medical device technologies is shaped partly by the medical frame, the healthcare sector to which products are geared. This in itself defines parameters which constrain the possible domestication, reinvention and resistance to particular technologies that users might be able to conceive. The case studies have shown that the development and deployment of medical devices reconfigures social and organisational relations, and social actors can reconfigure technologies to a greater or lesser degree, both in cycles of redesign and modification and in interpretation in the circumstances of their use. Key to the pathway of device technology/governance formations are the constructed, complex characteristics of the technology – including its mode of action upon the human body, its material and components and its linking in interdependent technology systems.

The key analytic issue here is the flexibility of technology. The case studies show tension between irreversibilities of lock-in and path dependence on the one hand, and flexibility of configuration in practice and interpretability on the other. Thus some technologies are configurational technologies, in which users build implementations that differ from set-up to set-up and are relatively open-ended (Fleck, 1994), while at the other end of the spectrum are 'discrete' technologies, which are in essence 'black-boxes' which are relatively impervious to user intervention. Alongside this distinction, I have distinguished between technologies in which usership involves a high degree of interpretation (PSA test) and those with a low 'affordance' (Hutchby, 2001) of interpretability (artificial hips). The analysis of devices suggests that not only is 'configurability' an important feature of the technology–social actor relationship, but also that 'interpretability' is crucial. Among the case studies considered here, infusion pumps are clearly a configurational technology, while the surgical technologies of orthopaedics and TE are discrete technologies with low configurability. However, a discrete device technology is not necessarily a 'low-interpretation' technology, as shown by the cases of the PSA test and the coagulometer.

Thus the sociality of medical device technology is variable between devices. Infusion pumps are highly 'social' but not in the sense that the PSA test is. In the PSA case the sociality of the technology lies in the simplicity of the material technology *per se* allied with the extreme uncertainty of its usership in the production and meaningful social interpretation of its 'outputs'. In the case of infusion pumps, on the other hand, the sociality of the technology lies in the complex nexus of medico-social and medico-organisational relationships in which a functionally complex device is deployed, a sociality whose nature will change with the increasing incorporation of ICT features.

Users may be 'configured' through alignment with specific technicalities of devices, as I have mentioned in the case of the privatisation of knowledge related to hips and pumps. Thus the clustering of interdependent technologies illustrated by infusion pump networking and smart customisable safety-related rules creates lock-in. Hips, infusion pumps and coagulometers 'require' training on the part of users, an explicit form of configuring the user as a competent actor for the technology. User training, either by state agency or by manufacturer, is to the fore with the coagulometer, hip prosthesis and the infusion pump, but in the case of the PSA test, the 'training' – the negotiation of a relationship of user to technology – takes the form of information provision and counselling. This is predicated on the highly uncertain interpretability of the technology – in medical terms. PSA testing inhabits a space on the cusp of society and the healthcare system, making for acute interpretative dilemmas for social actors who are presented with the opportunity to adopt the technology in healthcare practice and as part of subjective identities.

So some medical devices are 'more social' and 'more interpretable' than others. This final discussion has shown that for each device there is a different balance of forces between 'social' shaping and 'technological' shaping. While the concept of co-construction or co-production can be used to encapsulate this analysis, it does little to illuminate it. In this book I have examined the dynamics of innovation and governation of selected device technologies and have analysed them in terms of the conundrum of society/technology. In the spirit of the 'technology-in-practice' approach (Timmermans & Berg, 2003a), I have looked at technologies that are not high profile in the public sphere. Focusing on such more or less unexceptional devices has enabled an analysis of the dynamic movements of innovation, governation and usership which interact with their artefactual technology in and around the constraints of the healthcare sector. The inescapable conclusion of this analysis is that generalisations about the relationship between medical technology and society must be very carefully scrutinised with empirical evidence, and that the dynamic relationship between the specifics of a medical device technology and the specifics of a social process takes distinctive forms.

Notes

1 Innovation, Evidence and Governance of Medical Technology

1. Bijker's concept of 'technological frame' is that 'frames' govern the way that people/social groups relate to and act towards technology. It can apply to both production and use of technology. Frames are both enabling and constraining, enabling by constituting resources and organisation, limiting the range of possibilities for development. A frame can include, for example, current theory, test procedures, users' practices, core goals/problems of the developer, cultural beliefs or values and tacit knowledge (Bijker, 1994). A criticism of the concept concerns the origin, durability and extent of frames in relation to particular technologies – for example, the organisation of many medical specialties is highly resilient in the face of innovative medical devices (Hyysalo, 2004).
2. Under the conditions of 'mode 2' knowledge production (Gibbons et al., 1994) and 'post-normal science' (Funtowicz and Ravetz, 1992) the relationship between science and policy is changing.

2 Approaching Technology

1. I use Barry's (2001; 2006) concept of a 'technological zone' here in a fairly loose way. I do not have the space to discuss or develop the concept in detail (this is the subject of a separate project). A 'technological zone' (Barry gives high energy physics as an example) may comprise linked organisations, expertise, technical standards, patents, material technology, production methods, inventors, scientists, policymakers, users and so on. The concept, as a start, can be conceived of being as more focused and technology-specific than a product-defined 'sector' and also as cross-cutting conventional sectors and national jurisdictions.

3 The World of Medical Devices

1. Throughout the book, I refer broadly to 'the UK' as the main focus of the analysis. In fact, aspects of the devolution of governmental health policy within the UK – between England, Scotland, Wales and Northern Ireland – mean that when discussing the jurisdiction of, especially, particular regulatory bodies, the correct reference would in fact be sometimes to England only, sometimes to England and Wales only, and sometimes to the four countries. Because these differences are not central to the thread of my discussion, I have ignored them in most instances.

4 Artificial Hips: The Surveillance of Success

1. The story of Charnley has been recounted in a hagiographic biography (Waugh, 1990), and the interesting social and institutional pedigree of orthopaedics peculiar to North West England, to which Charnley's work may be traced, has also been documented (Pickstone, 2006).
2. For fuller accounts of the recent history of innovation in design and materials, see Faulkner (2002) and Neary (2007). An orthopaedic insider's account of the early history is in Scales (1965).
3. I was told by a senior member of NICE, in a research interview, that the 3-year criterion was justified because the failure rate of the device was usually linear and therefore three years was a good predictor of ten years' performance. Other European countries' orthopaedic communities, such as Norway, however, felt that the 3-year criterion was too weak.
4. Technical standards include EN12010 1998: Non-active surgical implants – Joint replacement implants – Particular requirements; EN12563: Non-active surgical implants – Joint replacement implants – Specific requirements for hip joint replacement implants. See CEN TC285 (Technical Committee 285) for relevant work programme and other standards.

5 The PSA Test for Prostate Cancer: Risk Constructs Governance?

1. DIPEx is a UK-based online resource that collects and comments on citizens' experiences in the form of video and audio testimonies elicited by interviewing, of an increasingly wide range of diseases and the processes of their diagnosis and treatment. It was created by the Division of Public Health & Primary Health Care at the University of Oxford as a facility that enables patients and prospective patients to see and hear people giving accounts of their own experiences. It is used as a teaching resource as well as a social support facility, and has won an award for social innovation.

6 Infusion Pumps: Usership and the Governance of Error

1. The work contributed to Mara Souza's PhD thesis at Federal University of Bahia, Salvador, Brazil (Souza, 2007).
2. In the US, leading technology assessment organisation ECRI has recently deemed non-smart infusion pumps, that is, without dose-error reduction software, to be unacceptable.
3. It is tempting to compare the 'guessability' level with the usability of mobile phones as well as video recorders.
4. Collaborative Procurement Hubs: recent reorganisation of NHS procurement process in the UK aimed at enabling coordinated regional procurement, contracts. See also Chapter 3.

7   Coagulometers: Healthcare Governance at Home

1. The two founders of Goldshield (among several other pharmaceutical companies selling antibiotic products to the NHS) were the subjects of a major UK Serious Fraud Office criminal investigation and a Department of Health lawsuit in the early 2000s into price-fixing and a market-sharing cartel for Marevan/warfarin drugs between 1996 and 2000. They were charged with conspiracy to defraud the NHS at a court hearing in 2006. In spite of refuting the charges, the company made several million-pound payments to the Department of Health in out of court settlement and the two founders resigned in 2007. At the time of writing, the criminal hearing was due in 2008.
2. The following website lists over 100 different brand names for warfarin, many of which are explicit in representing its common public identity as 'rat-poison': http://www.mongabay.com/health/medications/Warfarin.html, accessed May 2007.
3. One of the connections between the case studies of devices described in this book is that in 1990 German company Boehringer Mannheim purchased English engineering company Charles F. Thackray Ltd. in Leeds, England. As noted, Thackrays was the original manufacturer of the Charnley hip described in Chapter 4 of this book. The acquisition could be regarded as bringing together two of the world's leading manufacturers of total hip replacements. In 1998 Roche became the parent company of Depuy, by then the owner of Thackrays.
4. saferhealthcare is an online resource based in the UK and developed by the NPSA, BMJ Publishing Group and the Institute for Healthcare Improvement.
5. The extent of near-patient and self-monitoring policies and practices across the healthcare providers of the UK is currently unknown.

8   Device or drug? Governation of Tissue Engineering

1. See Chapter 2, note 1.
2. I gratefully acknowledge the support of the Economic and Social Research Council, via awards L218252058 and RES-000-22-1814, and the support of research team members Julie Kent, Ingrid Geesink, David FitzPatrick and Peter Glasner in this work.
3. Lexicographically, this term combines 'governance' with 'innovation' to convey the dynamic interdependence of the two concepts. The 'governation' term is similar in intention to the concept of 'innofusion' that has been coined to suggest the interdependence of technological innovation and diffusion processes (Fleck, 1988).

Bibliography

Abraham J. and Lewis G. (2000) *Regulating medicines in Europe: Competition, expertise and public health.* London: Routledge.

Abraham, J. and Lewis, G. (2002) 'Citizenship, Medical Expertise and the Capitalist Regulatory State in Europe', *Sociology*, 36 (1): 67–88.

Abraham, J. and Davis, C. (2007) 'Interpellative Sociology of Pharmaceuticals: Problems and Challenges for Innovation and Regulation in the 21st Century', *Technology Analysis & Strategic Management*, 19 (3): 387–402.

Advisory Group on Health Technology Assessment. (ca. 1992) *Assessing the effects of health technologies: Principles–practice–proposals.* London: Department of Health (undated).

Altenstetter C. (1996) 'Regulating healthcare technologies and medical supplies in the European Economic Area', *Health Policy*, 35: 33–52.

Altenstetter, C. (2004) *Regulatory Governance of Medical Devices in the European Union: Beyond Theories of European Integration.* Fifth European Conference on Health Economics, London 2004, 8–11 September. <http://www.lse.ac.uk/collections/LSEHealthAndSocialCare/>.Accessed 5 December 2006.

Anderson, J., Neary, N. and Pickstone, J. (2007) *Surgeons, Manufacturers and Patients: A Transatlantic History of Total Hip Replacement.* Basingstoke: Palgrave Macmillan.

Anon. (2004) 'Self-testing is favourite', *Medical Device Technology*, May 2004, 6.

Anon. (2007) *Orthopaedic tissue re-engineering.* http://leva.leeds.ac.uk/res-group/biomedical/biomedical.html. University of Leeds. Accessed October 2007.

Ansell, J. (2007) *Self-management of oral anticoagulation.* http://www.clotcare.com/. Accessed November 2007.

Ansell, J., Jacobson, A., Levy, J., Voller, H. and Hasenkam, J. M. (2005) 'Guidelines for implementation of patient self-testing and patient self-management of oral anticoagulation. International consensus guidelines prepared by International Self-Monitoring Association for Oral Anticoagulation'. *International Journal of Cardiology*, 99: 37–45.

Anticoagulation Europe (ACE). (2007) *About self-testing.* http://www.anticoagulationeurope.org/selftesting.html. Accessed June 2006.

ANVISA. (2004) Boletim informativo de Tecnovigilância: riscos associados ao uso de bombas de infusão. Brazil: Agência Nacional de Vigilância Sanitária, <http://www.anvisa.gov.br/divulga/public/tecnovigilancia/bit/2004/07_04.pdf>. Accessed 3 August 2006.

Apkon, M., Leonard, J., Probst, L., DeLizio, L. and Vitale, R. (2004) 'Design of a safer approach to intravenous drug infusions: failure mode effects analysis', *Quality and Safety in Health Care*, 13: 265–71.

Association of British Healthcare Industries (ABHI). (2002) *A Competitiveness Analysis of the Healthcare Industry in the United Kingdom.* London: Association of British Health Care Industries.

Atiyeh, B. S., Hayek, S. N. and Gunn, S. W. (2005) 'New technologies for burn wound closure and healing—Review of the literature', *Burns*, 31 (8): 944–56.

213

Balas, E. A. and Iakovidis, I. (1999) 'Distance technologies for patient monitoring', *British Medical Journal*, 319, 1309-U82.

Ballard, K. and Elston, MA. (2005) 'Medicalization: a multidimensional concept', *Social Theory and Health*, 3 (3): 229–41.

Barach, P. (2002) 'Lessons from the USA', in Emslie, Knox, Pickstone (eds).

Barad, K. (1998) 'Getting real: technoscientific practices and the materialization of reality', *Differences: A Journal of Feminist Cultural Studies* 10: 88–128.

Barry, A. (2001) *Political machines: governing a technological society*. London: Athlone Press.

Barry, A. (2006) 'Technological Zones', *European Journal of Social Theory*, 9 (2): 239–53.

Bath Institute of Medical Engineering. (2003) *Volumetric pump: Fresenius Vial MVP+ MS*. Bath: Medicines and Healthcare products Regulatory Agency.

Battista, R. N. (2006) 'Expanding the scientific basis of health technology assessment: A research agenda for the next decade', *International Journal of Technology Assessment in Health Care*, 22 (3): 275–80.

Baxterhealthcare. (2006) *Baxter & Patient Safety*, www.baxterhealthcare.co.uk/. Accessed November 2007.

BBC. (2004) Corcern over hip replacement ops. <http://news.bbc.co.uk/1/hi/health/3683847.stm>. Accessed August 2007.

BBC2. (1993) *The High Price Of Hips*. BBC Television programme, 26 February.

BBC Radio 4. '*Am I Normal?*' Series 2. Cancer. 14 November 2006. http://www.bbc.co.uk/radio4/science/am_i_normal_series_2.html. Accessed August 2007.

Beck, U. (1992) *Risk society: Towards a new modernity*. London: Sage Publications.

Berger, P. L. and Luckmann, T. (1967) *The social construction of reality. A treatise in the sociology of knowledge*. London: Allen Lane, The Penguin Press.

Beyth, R. J. (2005) 'Patient self-management of anticoagulation: An idea whose time has come', *Annals of Internal Medicine*, 142: 73–4.

Bhavnani, M. and Shiach, C. R. (2002) 'Patient self-management of oral anticoagulation', *Clinical and Laboratory Haematology*, 24: 253–7.

Bijker, W. E. (1995) *Of bicycles, Bakelite, and bulbs: Toward a theory of sociotechnical change*. Cambridge, MA; London: MIT Press.

Bijker, W. E., Hughes, T. P. and Pinch, T. J. (1987) *The social construction of technological systems: New directions in the sociology and history of technology*. Cambridge, MA; London, MIT Press.

Biomet. (1999) Hip systems. <http://www.biomet.com/surgeons/product/hips.html>. Accessed July 2003.

Black, I. (2001) EC safety moves over silicone breast implants. *The Guardian*, 22 March, <www.guardian.co.uk>.

Bloor, M. (2001) 'On the consulting room couch with citizen science: a consideration of the sociology of scientific knowledge perspective on practitioner-patient relationships', *Medical Sociology News*, 27 (3): 19–40.

Blume, S. S. (1992) *Insight and Industry: On the Dynamics of Technological Change in Medicine*. Cambridge MA: MIT Press.

Blume, S. S. (1995) 'Cochlear implantation: Establishing clinical feasibility, 1957–1982', in N. Rosenberg, A. Gelijns, and H. Dawkins (eds), *Sources of medical technology, Medical innovation at the crossroads*, vol. 5. (pp. 97–124). Washington, DC: Institute of Medicine/National Academy of Sciences.

Blume, S. S. (1997) 'The Rhetoric and Counter-Rhetoric of a "Bionic" Technology', *Science, Technology, & Human Values*, 22 (1): 31–56.

Bock, A. K., Ibarreta, D. and Rodriguez-Cerezo, E. (2003) *Human tissue-engineered products: Today's market and future prospects*—synthesis report EUR 21000 EN. Institute for Prospective Technological Studies IPTS and Joint Research Centre EC.

Bodewitz, H. J. H. W., Buurma, H. and de Vries, G. H. (1987) 'Regulatory science and the social management of trust in medicine', in W. E. Bijker, T. P. Hughes and T. Pinch (eds), *The social construction of technological systems: New directions in the sociology and history of technology* (pp. 243–59). Cambridge, MA; London: MIT Press.

Booth, R. E. (1994) 'Current concepts in joint replacement: The closing circle: Limitations of total joint arthroplasty', *Orthopedics*, 17 (9): 157–159.

Bowker, G. C. and Leigh Star, S. (1999) *Sorting things out: Classification and its consequences.* Cambridge: MIT Press.

Brett J., Watson E., Hewitson P., Bukach C., Edwards A., Elwyn G. and Austoker J. (2005). 'PSA testing for prostate cancer: an online survey of the views and reported practice of General Practitioners in the UK', *BMC Family Practice*, 6: 24.

Brindle L. A., Oliver S. E., Dedman D., Donovan J. L., Neal D. E., Hamdy F. C., Lane J. A. and Peters T. J. (2006). 'Measuring the psychosocial impact of population-based prostate-specific antigen testing for prostate cancer in the UK', *BJU International* 98 (4): 777–82.

British Orthopaedic Association (BOA). (1999) *Total hip replacement: A guide to best practice.* BOA, London.

Brown, A., Wells, P., Jaffey, J., McGahan, L., Poon, M.-C., Cimon, K. and Campbell, K. (2007) *Devices for point-of-care monitoring of long-term oral anticoagulation therapy: clinical and cost effectiveness.* Ottawa: Canadian Agency for Drugs and Technologies in Health.

Brown, N. and Michael, M. (2003) 'A Sociology of Expectations: Retrospecting Prospects and Prospecting Retrospects', *Technology Analysis and Strategic Management*, 15 (1): 3–18.

Brown, N., and Webster, A. (2004) *New medical technologies and society: Re-ordering life.* Cambridge: Polity Press.

Brown, N., Faulkner, A., Kent, J. and Michael, M. (2006) 'Regulating hybrids – "cleaning up" and "making a mess" in tissue engineering and transpecies transplantation', *Social Theory and Health*, 4 (1): 1–24.

Bud R. (1999) 'In the engine of industry: regulators of biotechnology, 1970–86', in M. Bauer (ed.). *Resistance to new technology: Nuclear power, information technology and biotechnology* (pp. 293–310). Cambridge: Cambridge University Press.

Bulstrode, C. J. K., Murray, D. W., Carr, A. J., Pynsent, P. B., and Carter S. R. (1993) 'Designer Hips', *British Medical Journal*, 306: 732–3.

Bulstrode C. (1996) 'Total hip replacement: the way forward', *Annals of the Royal College of Surgeons of England* 78 (2): 129–32.

Callon, M. (1986) 'The sociology of an actor network: the case of the electric vehicle', in M. Callon, J. Law and A. Rip (eds), *Mapping the dynamics of science and technology: sociology of science in the real world* (pp. 19–34). London: Macmillan.

Callon, M. (2004) 'Europe wrestling with technology', *Economy and Society*, 33 (1): 121–34.

Callon, M. and Rabeharisoa, V. (2003) 'Research "in the wild" and the shaping of new social identities', *Technology in Society*, 25 (2): 193–204.

Cameron E., and Bernardes J. (1998) 'Gender and disadvantage in health: men's health for a change', *Sociology of Health and Illness*, 20 (5): 673–93.

Cardinal Health. (2007) <www.cardinal.com/alaris>. Accessed October 2007

Catalona, W. J. and Maggiore, J. A. (2005) PSA and Free-PSA Testing for Prostate Cancer Is Still a Lifesaver (Catalona et al., 2005). Clinical Lab Products, February 2005.

CEN. (2001) *About CEN and European Standardisation*, CHeF Healthcare Forum Mission, <http://www.cenorm.be.htm>. Accessed April 2001.

Centre for Evidence-based Purchasing (CEP). (2007) *Evaluation Report Hospira Plum A+ Volumetric Infusion Pump*, CEP 07014, <www.pasa.nhs.uk>. Accessed November 2007.

Chamberlain J., Melia J., Moss S. and Brown J. (1997) 'The diagnosis, management, treatment and costs of prostate cancer in England and Wales', *Health Technology Assessment*, 1 (3) (whole volume).

Chapple A., Ziebland S., Shepperd S., Miller R., Herxheimer A. and McPherson A. (2002) 'Why men with prostate cancer want wider access to prostate specific antigen testing: qualitative study', *British Medical Journal*, 325: 737–41.

Chignon, T. (2003) *Initiatives to Harmonize Regulations of Human Tissue/Cell Products in the European Union*, <http://www.raps.org.rainteractive>. Accessed January 2003.

Christensen, C. M., and Overdorf, M. (2000) 'Meeting the Challenge of Disruptive Change', *Harvard Business Review*, March-April 2000.

Clar, C., Cummins, E., McIntyre, L., Thomas, S., Lamb, J., Bain, L., Jobanputra, P. and Waugh, N. (2004) *Clinical and cost-effectiveness of autologous chondrocyte implantation for cartilage defects in knee joints; Technology assessment report*. Aberdeen Health Technology Assessment Group, University of Aberdeen.

Clarke, A. E., Shim, J. K., Mamo, L., Fosket, J. R. and Fishman, J. R. (2003) 'Biomedicalization: Technoscientific transformations of health, illness, and U.S. biomedicine', *American Sociological Review*, 68 (2): 161–94.

Concato, J., Wells, C. K., Horwitz, R. I., Penson, D., Fincke, G., Berlowitz, D. R., Froehlich, G., Blake, D., Vickers, M. A., Gehr, G. A., Raheb, N. H., Sullivan, G. and Peduzzi, P. (2006) 'The effectiveness of screening for prostate cancer – A nested case-control study', *Archives of Internal Medicine*, 166: 38–43.

Collingridge, D. (1980) *The social control of technology*. London: Frances Pinter Publishers.

Collins, H. M. and Pinch, T. J. (1998) *The golem at large: what you should know about technology*. Cambridge: Cambridge University Press.

Committee on the Safety of Devices (CSD). (2004) *Minutes of Meeting 1 July 2004* <http://www.mhra.gov.uk/>. Accessed February 2006.

Conrad, P. (2005) 'The shifting engines of medicalization', *Journal of Health and Social Behaviour*, 46: 3–14.

Cookson, R. and Hutton, J. (2003) 'Regulating the economic evaluation of pharmaceuticals and medical devices: A European perspective', *Health Policy* 63 (2): 167–78.

Consumers Association. (2002) 'Don't Try These At Home: Home Testing Kits', *Health Which?* 10–13.

Consumers Association. (1997) Hip replacements. *Health Which?* February 1997: 32–3.

Cosmi, B., Palareti, G., Moia, M., Carpenedo, M., Pengo, V., Biasiolo, A., Rampazzo, P., Morstabilini, G. and Testa, S. (2000) 'Assessment of patient capability to self-adjust oral anticoagulant dose: a multicenter study on home use of a portable prothrombin time monitor (COAGUCHECK)', *Haematologica*, 85: 826–31.

Cox, M., and Tinkler, J. (2000) 'Biomaterials regulation: innovative products – outgrowing the European Framework?' *Action in Biomaterials*, Issue 4, May 2000, The Biomaterials Partnership.

Council of the European Union. (2007) *Proposal for a Regulation of the European Parliament and of the Council on advanced therapy medicinal products and amending Directive 2001/83/EC and Regulation (EC) No 726/2004 – Political Agreement*, General Secretariat of the Council, Strasbourg.

Cromheecke, M. E., Levi, M., Colly, L. P., de Mol, B. J. M., Prins, M. H., Hutten, B. A., Mak, R., Keyzers, K. C. J. and Buller, H. R. (2000) 'Oral anticoagulation self-management and management by a specialist anticoagulation clinic: a randomised cross-over comparison', *Lancet*, 356: 97–102.

Datamonitor. (2005) 'Healthcare Equipment and Supplies in Europe: Industry Profile', New York, London: Datamonitor plc.

Datamonitor. (2006) 'Healthcare Equipment and Supplies in The United Kingdom: Industry Profile', May 2006. New York, London: Datamonitor plc.

Davey, C. (2003a) *Syringe pump: Medex Medfusion 3500*. Bath: Bath Institute of Medical Engineering.

Davey, C. (2003b) *Volumetric pump: Baxter Colleague 3*. Bath: Bath Institute of Medical Engineering.

Davey, C. (2005) *Target controlled infusion (TCI) systems part one: Diprifusor pumps*. Bath: Bath Institute of Medical Engineering.

Davidson, K. and Barber, V. (2004) Electronic monitoring of patients in general wards. *Nursing Standard*, 18 (49): 42–6.

Davies, E. and Evans, G. (1999) '3M Capital of Hip Replacements: The Isle of Wight experience', *Clinical Risk*, 5 (4): 115–9.

Davison, C., Smith, G. D. and Frankel, S. (1991) 'Lay epidemiology and the prevention paradox – the implications of coronary candidacy for health-education', *Sociology of Health & Illness*, 13 (1): 1–19.

Dawson, J., Fitzpatrick, R., Carr, A. and Murray, D. (1996) 'Questionnaire on the perceptions of patients about total hip replacement', *Journal of Bone and Joint Surgery*, 78-B: 185–90.

Dearnaley, D. P., Kirby, R. S., Kirk, D., Malone, P., Simpson, R. J. and Williams, G. (1999) 'Diagnosis and management of early prostate cancer. Report of a British Association of Urological Surgeons (BAUS) Working Party', *BJU International*, 83, 18–33.

Delanty, G. and Rumford, C. (2005) *Rethinking Europe: Social theory and the implications of Europeanization*. London: Routledge.

Department of Health. (2000) *National joint replacement registry. A consultation document*. London: Department of Health.

Department of Health. (2001a) *The expert patient: A new approach to chronic disease management for the 21st century*. London: Department of Health.

Department of Health. (2001b) *A Code of Practice for Tissue Banks providing tissues of human origin for therapeutic purposes*. London: Department of Health.

Department of Health. (2004) *Building a safer NHS for patients – improving medication safety*. London: Department of Health. <www.doh.gov.uk/buildsafenhs/medicationsafety>.

Department of Health Expert Group. (2000) *An Organisation with a Memory: Report of an expert group on learning from adverse events in the NHS, chaired by the Chief Medical Officer*. London: The Stationery Office.

Department of Health, Carruthers, I., and Philip, P. (2006) 'Safety first: A report for patients, clinicians and healthcare managers', Department of Health, London. <http://www.dh.gov.uk/en/Publicationsandstatistics/>. Accessed November 2007.

DePuy. (1997) *Annual Report*. DePuy International Ltd, Leeds.

Dickenson, J. E. (1983) 'Syringe pumps', *British Journal of Hospital Medicine*, 187–91.

Donovan, J. (1997) *Interviews with orthopaedic surgeons about hip replacement*. Unpublished report, Department of Social Medicine, University of Bristol.

Donovan, J. L., Frankel, S., Faulkner, A., Gillatt, D. and Hamdy, F. C. (1999) 'Dilemmas in treating early prostate cancer: The evidence and a questionnaire survey of consultant urologists in the UK', *British Medical Journal*, 318: 299–300.

Donovan, J. L., Frankel, S. J., Neal, D. E. and Hamdy, F. C. (2001) 'Screening for prostate cancer in the UK', *British Medical Journal*, 323: 763–4.

Donovan, J., Mills, N., Smith, M., Brindle, L., Jacoby, A., Peters, T., Frankel, S., Neal, D., Hamdy, F. and Little, P. (2002) 'Quality improvement report: Improving design and conduct of randomised trials by embedding them in qualitative research: ProtecT (prostate testing for cancer and treatment) study', *British Medical Journal*, 325: 766–70.

Donovan, J., Hamdy, F., Neal, D., Peters, T., Oliver, S., Brindle, L., Jewell, D., Powell, P., Gillatt, D., Dedman, D., Mills, N., Smith, M., Noble, S. and Lane, A. (2003) 'Prostate Testing for Cancer and Treatment (ProtecT) feasibility study', *Health Technology Assessment*, 7, 14 (whole volume).

DTI. (2005) *UK Sector Competitiveness: Analysis of six healthcare equipment sectors*. Department of Trade and Industry, London.

Dunn, T. (2004a) *Alaris Asena GW: Volumetric pump*. Bath: Bath Institute of Medical Engineering.

Dunn, T. (2004b) *Dose limiting software for infusion devices*. Bath: Bath Institute of Medical Engineering.

Dunn, T., Davey, C., and Lipson, M. (2006) *Investigating a new method of usability testing to help inform purchasing policy within the NHS*, http://people.bath.ac.uk/mpscd/pumpPages/. Accessed 15 November 2007.

Dunn, T. (2006) 'How infusion pumps work', in *Pumps in practice: seminar and training day*. Anais; London: Medicines and Healthcare products Regulatory Agency.

EC DG Enterprise. (2001) *Guidelines for the classification of medical devices*. Brussels: European Commission.

EC DG Enterprise. (2002) *Need for a legislative framework for human tissue engineered products*, http://europa.eu.int/comm/enterprise/medical_devices/consult_tissue_engineer.htm. Accessed July 2002.

EC DG Enterprise. (2004a) *Proposal for a harmonised regulatory framework on human tissue engineered products*. DG Enterprise, European Commission, Brussels.

EC DG Enterprise. (2004b) *Proposal for a harmonised regulatory framework on human tissue engineered products. Summary of contributions.* April 2004, Brussels.

EC DG Enterprise. (2004c) *Proposal for a harmonised regulatory framework on human tissue engineered products: DG Enterprise Consultation Paper*, 6 April 2004. Presented at Stakeholders' Conference, 16 April 2004, Brussels.

EC DG Enterprise & Industry. (2005) *Proposal for a regulation of the European Parliament and of the Council on advanced therapy medicinal products and amending Directive 2001/83/EC and Regulation (EC) No 726/2004.* 2005/0227(COD). 16 November 2005, European Commission, Brussels.

EC DG Enterprise & Industry. (2007) *Guidelines on a medical devices vigilance system*, MEDDEV 2.12-1 rev 5, Brussels, European Commission. http://ec.europa.eu/enterprise/medical_devices/meddev/2_12_1-rev_5-2007-fin2.pdf. Accessed November 2007.

Edwards, R. H. T. (1999) 'Is it time for an Illich Collaboration to make available information on the harms of medical care?', *British Medical Journal*, 318: 58 [Letter].

Emslie, S., Knox, K. and Pickstone, M. (eds). (2002) *Improving patient safety: insights from American, Australian and British health care.* Based on the proceedings of a joint ECRI and Department of Health conference to introduce the National Patient Safety Agency. Welwyn Garden City, ECRI Europe.

Enoch, S., Shaaban, H. and Dunn, K. W. (2005) 'Informed consent should be obtained from patients to use products (skin substitutes) and dressings containing biological material', *Journal of Medical Ethics*, 31: 2–6.

Epstein, S. (1996), *Impure science: Aids, activism, and the politics of knowledge*, Berkeley, London: University of California Press.

Epstein, S. (2000) 'RePlacing citizenship: AIDS activism and radical democracy', *Isis*, 91 (2): 423–4.

Essink Bot, M. L., de Koning, H. J., Nijs, H. G., Kirkels, W. J., van der Maas, P. J. and Schroder, F. H. (1998) 'Short-term effects of population based screening for prostate cancer on health-related quality of life', *Journal of the National Cancer Institute*, 90: 925–31.

Etzkowitz, H. and Leydesdorff, L. (2000) 'The dynamics of innovation: from national systems and "Mode 2" to a Triple Helix of university industry government relations', *Research Policy*, 29 (2): 109–23.

Eucomed. (2007a) 'Musculoskeletal health: Advances in medical technology: porous orthopaedic implants', *Medical Technology Focus* Issue 60 – May/June 2007.

Eucomed. (2007b) *Eucomed Position on the Advanced Therapy Medicinal Products Commission Proposal* COM (2005) 567 Final 2005/0227 (COD), <www.eucomed.org>. Accessed November 2007.

Eucomed. (2007c) *European Med Tech Industry: Eucomed Publishes New Industry Brief*, <www.eucomed.org>. Accessed April 2007.

Eucomed. (2008) 'Infusion pumps', <www.eucomed.org> (Forthcoming).

EuropaBio. (2002) *Need for a legislative framework for human tissue engineering and tissue-engineered products – EuropaBio position paper.* <http://www.europabio.org/>. Accessed November 2007.

European Association of Tissue Banks (EATB). (2005) *Comments on DG Enterprise Proposal to Regulate Tissue Engineered Products*. http://ec.europa.eu/enterprise/ pharmaceuticals/advtherapies/ stakehcom2005/. Accessed July 2006.

European Commission. (2003) Commission Directive 2003/63/EC, amending Directive 2001/83/EC of the European Parliament and of the Council on the Community code relating to medicinal products for human use. *Official Journal of the European Union*, L158: 46–94. Accessed June 2003.

European Commission (EC). (2005) *Proposal for a regulation of the European Parliament and of the Council on advanced therapy medicinal products and amending Directive 2001/83/EC and Regulation (EC) No 726/2004.* 2005/0227(COD). EC, Brussels 16 November 2005.

European Commission. (2005) Commission Directive 2005/50/EC of 11 August 2005 on the reclassification of hip, knee and shoulder joint replacements in the framework of Council Directive 93/42/EEC concerning medical devices (Text with EEA relevance). Commission Directive 2005/50/EC. 11 August 2005. *Official Journal* L 210, 12 August 2005: 0041–3.

European Commission DG Enterprise and Industry. (2007) *IVMDD labelling*. Brussels.

European Health Committee, Committee of Experts on Management of Safety and Quality in Health Care. (2005) *Prevention of adverse events in health care, a system approach*. Strasbourg: Council of Europe. http://www.simpatie.org/. Accessed November 2007.

European Parliament. (2003) *Human tissues and cells*, plenary debate, 9 April 2003 — Strasbourg, <www.europarl.europa.eu>. Accessed March 2004.

Evans, R., Edwards, A. G. K., Elwyn, G., Watson, E., Grol, R., Brett, J. and Austoker, J. (2007) '"It's a maybe test": men's experiences of prostate specific antigen testing in primary care'. *British Journal of General Practice*, 57: 303–10.

Faulkner, A. (1997) '"Strange bedfellows" in the laboratory of the NHS? An analysis of the new science of health technology assessment in the United Kingdom', in M. A. Elston (ed.) *The sociology of medical science and technology*. Sociology of Health and Illness Monograph No. 3, (pp. 183–207). Blackwell: Oxford.

Faulkner, A., Brookes, S. T., Donovan, J., Selley, S., Gillatt, D. and Hamdy, F. (2000) 'The use of prostate-specific antigen testing in the detection of local-ized prostate cancer: Current opinion and urological practice in the United Kingdom', *European Journal of Public Health*, 10: 289–95.

Faulkner, A., Kennedy, L. G., Baxter, K., Donovan, J., Wilkinson, M. and Bevan, G. (1998) 'Effectiveness of hip prostheses in primary total hip replacement: A critical review of evidence and an economic model', *Health Technology Assessment*, 2 (6): pp. i–iv, 1–134 (whole volume).

Faulkner, A. (2002) 'Casing the joint: the material development of artificial hips', in K. Ott, D. Serlin and S. Mihm (eds). (2002) *Artificial Parts, Practical Lives: modern histories of prosthetics*. New York University Press, pp. 199–226.

Faulkner, A. and Kent, J. (2001) 'Innovation and regulation in human implant technologies: developing comparative approaches', *Social Science & Medicine*, 53: 895–913.

Faulkner, A., Kent, J., Fitzpatrick, D. and Geesink, I. (2003) 'Human tissue engineered products—drugs or devices?' *British Medical Journal*, 326: 1159–60.

Faulkner, A., Kent, J., Geesink, I. and Fitzpatrick, D. (2006). 'Purity and the dangers of regenerative medicine: regulatory innovation of human tissue engineered technology', *Social Science & Medicine*, 63: 2277–88.

Faulkner, A. (2008) 'Regulatory policy as innovation: constructing rules of engagement of a technological zone for tissue engineering in the European Union', *Research Policy*, forthcoming.

Faulkner, A., Geesink, I., Kent, J. and FitzPatrick, D. (2008) 'Tissue-engineered technologies: scientific biomedicine, frames of risk and regulatory regime-building in Europe', *Science as Culture*, 17(2): 195–222.

Fechter, R. J. and Barba, J. J. (2004) 'Failure Mode Effect Analysis Applied to the Use of Infusion Pumps', *Engineering in Medicine and Biology Society*, 2 (1–5): 3496–99.

Fengo, B., Finazzi, G., Testa, S. and Tripodi, A. (2003) 'Self-testing and self-management of oral anticoagulation therapy: Consensus of the Italian Federation of Anticoagulation Clinics', *Haematologica*, 88.

Finsterer, J., Stollberger, C. and Hopmeier, P. (2000) 'Home-made anticoagulation monitor vs. CoaguCheck-Plus (R) monitoring of oral anticoagulation', *Thrombosis Research*, 98: 571–5.

Fitzpatrick, R., Shortall, E., Sculpher, M., Murray, D., Morris, R., Lodge, M., Dawson, J., Call, A., Britton, A. and Briggs, A. (1998) 'Primary total hip replacement surgery: a systematic review of outcomes and modelling of cost-effectiveness associated with different prostheses', *Health Technology Assessment*, 2, pp. i–iv, 1–64 (whole volume).

Fitzmaurice, D. A. and Machin, S. J. (2001) 'Recommendations for patients undertaking self management of oral anticoagulation', *British Medical Journal*, 323: 985–9.

Fitzmaurice, D. A., Murray, E. T., Hobbs, F. D. R. and MacCahon, D. (2004) 'Self-management of anticoagulation: a randomized trial (SMART)', *British Journal of Haematology*, 125 (Suppl.): 56.

Fitzmaurice, D. (2006) 'Oral Anticoagulation Control: The European Perspective', *Journal of Thrombosis and Thrombolysis*, 21: 95–100.

Fleck, J. (1988) *Innofusion or diffusation? The nature of technological developments in robotics*, Edinburgh PICT Working Paper, University of Edinburgh.

Fleck, J. (1994) 'Learning By Trying – The Implementation of Configurational Technology', *Research Policy*, 23 (6): 637–52.

Food and Drug Administration. (2004) Medical Device Recalls: Class 2 Recall – Model 8100 Series Medley Medication Safety System Pump Module. <http://www.accessdata.fda.gov/>. Accessed 26 March 2006.

Food and Drug Administration. (2005) Medical Device Recalls: Class 1 Recall – Colleague and Colleague CX Volumetric Infusion Pumps. <http://www.accessdata.fda.gov/>. Accessed 26 March 2006.

Foote, S. B. (1992) *Managing the medical arms race: innovation and public policy in the medical device industry*. Berkeley and Los Angeles: University of California Press.

Foucault, M., Martin, L. H., Gutman, H. and Hutton, P. H. (1988) *Technologies of the Self: A Seminar with Michel Foucault*. Amherst: University of Massachusetts Press.

Fox, N., Ward, K. and O'Rourke, A. (2007) 'A sociology of technology governance for the information age: The case of pharmaceuticals, consumer advertising and the Internet', *Sociology*, 40 (2): 315–34.

Freidson, E. (1986) *Professional powers: A study of the institutionalization of formal knowledge*. Chicago: University of Chicago Press.

Fujita, K., Makimoto, K. and Hotokebuchi, T. (2006) 'Qualitative study of osteoarthritis patients' experience before and after total hip arthroplasty in Japan', *Nursing & Health Sciences*, 8 (2): 81–7.

Funtowicz, S. and Ravetz, J. (1992). 'Risk management as a post-normal science', *Risk Analysis*, 12 (1): 95–7.

Furtado, J. (2001) A indústria de equipamentos médico-hospitalares: elementos para uma caracterização de sua dimensão internacional, in B. Negri & G. D. Giovanni (eds), *Brasil: radiografia da saúde*. Campinas-SP: UNICAMP.

Gabbay, J. and Walley, T. (2006) 'Introducing new health interventions', *British Medical Journal*, 332: 64–5.

Gabe, J., Kelleher, D. and Williams, G. (eds). (1994) *Challenging medicine*. London: Routledge.

Gadelha, C. A. G. (2003) O complexo industrial da saúde e a necessidade de um enfoque dinâmico na economia da saúde. *Ciência e saúde coletiva*, 8: 521–35.

Gadelha, C. A. G. (2004) Complexo Industrial da Saúde: desafios para uma política de inovação e desenvolvimento, in M. D. Saúde (ed.), *Saúde no Brasil: contribuições para a agenda de prioridades de pesquisa*. 1st ed. Brasília.

Gardiner, C., Machin, K., Mackie, I., Williams, S. and Cohen H. (2005) *Patient self-management using the Coaguchek S*. London: MHRA.

Gardiner, C., Williams, K., Mackie, I. J., Machin, S. J. and Cohen, H. (2006) 'Can oral anticoagulation be managed using telemedicine and patient self-testing? A pilot study', *Clinical and Laboratory Haematology*, 28: 122–5.

Garmer, K., Liljegren, E., Osvalder, A.-L. and Dahlman, S. (2002) 'Application of usability testing to the development of medical equipment. Usability testing of a frequently used infusion pump and a new user interface for an infusion pump developed with a human factors approach', *International Journal of Industrial Ergonomics*, 29 (3): 145–59.

Geels, F. W. (2005) 'From sectoral systems of innovation to socio-technical systems. Insights about dynamics and change from sociology and institutional theory', *Research Policy*, 33: 897–920.

Gelijns, A. C. (1990) 'Comparing the development of drugs, devices, and clinical procedures', in A. C. Gelijns (ed.), *Modern methods of clinical investigation, Medical innovation at the crossroads*, vol. 1, pp. 147–201. Washington, DC: National Academy Press.

Gibbons, M., et al. (1994) *The new production of knowledge: The dynamics of science and research in contemporary societies*. Newbury Park, CA.

Graham, F. and Clark, D. (2005) 'The syringe driver and the subcutaneous route in palliative care: the inventor, the history and the implications', *Journal of Pain and Symptom Management*, 29 (1): 32–40.

Grigoris P. and Hamblen D. (1998) 'The control of new prosthetic implants (Editorial)', *Journal of Bone and Joint Surgery [Br]*, 80-B: 941–3.

Hambidge, D. (2002) 'Self management is the future', *British Medical Journal*, 324: 486.

Haque, M. S. (2002) 'Globalization, New Political Economy, and Governance: A Third World Viewpoint', *Administrative Theory & Praxis*, 24 (1): 103–24.

Harrison, S. (1998) 'The politics of evidence-based medicine', *Policy and Politics*, 26 (1): 15–31.

Havelin, L. I., Espehaug, B. and Vollset, S. E. (1993) 'The Norwegian arthroplasty register: A survey of 17,444 hip replacements 1987–1990', *Acta Orthopaedica Scandinavica*, 64 (3): 245–51.

Healthcare Industries Task Force (HITF). (2007) *Innovation for health: Making a difference*. <http://www.dh.gov.uk>. Accessed November 2007.

Hellman, K. (1997) 'Bioartificial organs as outcomes of tissue engineering. Scientific and regulatory issues', *Annals of the New York Academy of Sciences*, 831: 1–9.

Heneghan, C., Alonso-Coello, P., Garcia-Alamino,J. M., Perera, R., Meats, E. and Glasziou, P. (2006) 'Self-monitoring of oral anticoagulation: a systematic review and meta-analysis', *Lancet*, 367: 404–11.

Heneghan, C., Perera, R., Fitzmaurice, D., Meats, E. and Glasziou, P. (2007) 'Assessing differential attrition in clinical trials: self-monitoring of oral anticoagulation and type II diabetes', *BMC Medical Research Methodology*, 7: 18. <http://www.biomedcentral.com/1471-2288/7/18>.

Hewitson, P. and Austoker, J. (2005) 'Part 2: Patient information, informed decision-making and the psycho-social impact of prostate-specific antigen testing', *BJU International* 95 (S3): 16–32.

Hill, A. (2003) *Syringe pump: Micrel medical devices micropump*. Bath: Bath Institute of Medical Engineering.

Hill, A. (2007) 'Cancer warning for stressed out men', *Observer*, September 2, <http://www.guardian.co.uk/uk/2007/sep/02/health.gender>. Accessed November 2007.

Hoeyer, K. (2007) 'Multiple ways of knowing the hip', Presentation at *Society for Social Studies of Science* Annual Conference, Montreal, 11 October 2007.

House of Commons European Scrutiny Committee. (2006) *Thirty-first Report of Session 2005–06*, 26 June 2006. London: The Stationery Office.

Howson, A. (1998) 'Surveillance, knowledge and risk: The embodied experience of cervical screening', *Health*, 2 (2): 195–215.

Hughes, T. P. (1983) *Networks of power: Electrification in Western society, 1880-1930*. Baltimore: Johns Hopkins University Press.

Hughes-Jones, S. (2006) *C257 – Guideline for Patient Self-Testing/Management of International Normalised Ratio (INR)*. Personal communication: North West Wales NHS Trust.

Huiskes, R. (1993) 'Failed innovation in total hip replacement. Diagnosis and proposals for a cure', *Acta Orthopaedica Scandinavica*, 64 (6): 699–716.

Husch, M., Sullivan, C., Rooney, D., Barnard, C., Fotis, M., Clarke, J. and Noskin, G. (2005) 'Insights from the sharp end of intravenous medication errors: implications for infusion pump technology', *Quality and Safety in Health Care*, 14: 80–6.

Hutchby, I. (2001) Technologies, Texts and Affordances, *Sociology*, 35: 441–56.

Hyysalo, S. (2004) *Uses of Innovation: Wristcare in the practices of engineers and elderly*. Helsinki: University of Helsinki.

Hyysalo, S. (2006) 'Representations of use and practice-bound imaginaries in automating the safety of the elderly', *Social Studies of Science*, 36 (4): 599–626.

Illich, I. (1975) *Limits to Medicine: Medical Nemesis, the Expropriation of Health*. London: Calder and Boyars.

Invest in Germany GMBH. (2005) *German medical technology: milestones and clusters*. <http://www.invest-in-germany.de/>. Accessed 10 August 2006.

Irwin, A. (1995). *Citizen science: a study of people, expertise and sustainable development*. London: Routledge.

Irwin, A., Rothstein, H., Yearley, S. and McCarthy, E. (1997) 'Regulatory science – towards a sociological framework', *Futures*, 29 (1): 17–31.

Jones, G. (2003) 'Procuring Safer Medicines', *Hospital Pharmacist*, 10 (11): 501–2.

Johnson, T. R., Zhang, J., Patel, V., Keselman, A., Tang, X., Brixey, J., Paige, D. and Turley, J. (2005) 'The role of patient safety in the device purchasing process', in *Advances in Patient Safety: From Research to Implementation*, K. Henriksen, J. B. Battles, E. Marks and D. I. Lewin (eds). Agency for Healthcare Research and Quality, Rockville, MD, pp. 341–52. <http://www.ahrq.gov/downloads/>.

Keating, P. and Cambrosio, A. (2006) 'Risk on trial: the interaction of innovation and risk in cancer clinical trials', in T. Schlich, and U. Tröhler (eds). *The risks of medical innovation: Risk perception and assessment in historical context*, pp. 225–41. Abingdon, New York: Routledge.

Kelman, J. (2007) 'Five years of self-management', <http://www.anticoagula tioneurope.org/johnkelman.html>. Accessed July 2007.

Kelleher, D., Gabe, J. and Williams, G. (eds). (2006) *Challenging Medicine*. London: Routledge.

Kennedy, A., Gately, C., Rogers, A. and EPP-Evaluation-Team. (2003) *Assessing the Process of Embedding EPP (Expert Patient Programme) in the NHS*. Universities of Manchester and York: National Primary Care R&D Centre.

Kent, J. (2003) 'Lay Experts and the Politics of Breast Implants', *Public Understanding of Science*, 12 (4): 403–21.

Kent, J. and Faulkner, A. (2002) 'Regulating human implant technologies in Europe – understanding the new era in medical device regulation', *Health, Risk & Society*, 4 (2): 190–209.

Kent, J., Faulkner, A., Geesink, I. and FitzPatrick, D. (2006) 'Towards Governance of Human Tissue Engineered Technologies in Europe: Framing the case for a new regulatory regime', *Technological Forecasting and Social Change*, 73: 41–60.

Kinnealey, E., Fishman, G., Sims, N., Cooper, J. and DeMonaco, H. (2003) *Infusion Pumps with "Drug Libraries" at The Point of Care – A Solution for Safer Drug Delivery*. <www.npsf.org/download/Kinnealey.pdf>. Accessed September 2007.

Klein, H. D. and Kleinman, D. L. (2002) 'The Social Construction of Technology: Structural Considerations', *Science, Technology, & Human Values*, 27 (1): 28–52.

Koertke, H. and Koerfer, R. (2001) 'International Standardized Ratio self management after mechanical heart valve replacement: is an early start advantageous?', *Annals of Thoracic Surgery*, 72: 44–8.

Koertke, H., Zittermann, A., Mommertz, S., El-Arousy, M., Litmathe, J. and Koerfer, R. (2005) 'The Bad Oeynhausen concept of INR self-management', *Journal of Thrombosis and Thrombolysis*, 19: 25–31.

Langer, R. and Vacanti, J. P. (1993) 'Tissue engineering', *Science*, 260: 920–6.

Laupacis, A., Rorabeck, C. H., Bourne, R. B., Feeny, D., Tugwell, P. and Sim, D. A. (1989) 'Randomized trial in orthopedics: why, how and when?', *Journal of Bone and Joint Surgery*, 71-A (4): 555–63.

Law, J. (1987) 'Technology and heterogeneous engineering: the case of Portuguese expansion', *The social construction of technological systems*. Cambridge, MA: MIT Press.

Law, J., and Hassard, J. (eds). (1999) *Actor-network theory and after*. Oxford: Blackwell.

LeFanu, J. (2000) *The rise and fall of modern medicine*. London: Little Brown.

Lefever, J. (2006) 'What do adverse incidents tell us about infusion pumps?', in *IPumps in practice: seminar and training day*. Anais. London: Medicines and Healthcare products Regulatory Agency.

Lehoux, P. (2006) *The problem of health technology: policy implications for modern health care systems*, New York: Routledge.

Lehoux, P., and Blume, S. S. (2000) 'Technology assessment and the sociopolitics of health technologies', *Journal of Health Policy, Politics and Law*, 25 (6): 1083–120.

Longair, I., Gardiner, C., Pescott, M. A., Mackie, I. J., Cohen, H. and Machin, S. J. (2005) Hemosense INRatio™. <:ttp://www.pasa.doh.gov.uk/>. London: Department of Health Evaluation Centre, PASA.

Lupton, D. (1995). *The imperative of health: Public health and the regulated body*. London: Sage.

Lysaght, M. J. and Hazlehurst, A. L. (2004) 'Tissue engineering: The end of the beginning', *Tissue Engineering*, 10 (1–2): 309–20.

Lysaght, M. (2006) 'The Pathway to a Tissue Engineering Industry: Lessons from other transformational biotechnologies', Presentation at conference *Commercialisation of Tissue Engineering and Regenerative Medicine*, London, November 2006.

MacKenzie, D. A. and Wajcman, J. (eds). (1985) *The social shaping of technology: How the refrigerator got its hum*. Milton Keynes: Open University Press.

MacKenzie, D. A. (1999) 'Theories of technology and the abolition of nuclear weapons', in D. MacKenzie and J. Wajcman (eds). *The social shaping of technology*. Buckingham: Open University Press, Second Edition, pp. 419–42.

MacKenzie, D. A. and Wajcman, J. (1999) 'Introductory essay: the social shaping of technology', in D. A. MacKenzie and J. Wajcman (eds). *The social shaping of technology*, pp. 3–27.

Majone, G. (1997) 'The new European agencies: regulation by information', *European Journal of Public Policy*, 4 (2): 262–75.

Malerba, F. (2004) 'Sectoral systems of innovation: basic concepts', in F. Malerba, (ed.) *Sectoral systems of innovation: concepts, issues and analyses of six major sectors in Europe*. Cambridge: Cambridge University Press, pp. 9–41.

Malerba, F. (2006) 'Innovation in sectoral systems: What we know ... and what we would like to know', Presentation to *SPRU 40th Anniversary Conference*, University of Sussex.

Marcuse, H. (1964) *One-dimensional man: Studies in the ideology of advanced industrial society*, London: Ark.

Massoud, S. N., Hunter, J. B., Holdsworth, B. J., Wallace, W. A., and Juliusson, R. (1997) 'Early femoral loosening in one design of cemented hip replacement', *Journal of Bone & Joint Surgery – British*. Vol. 79 (4): 603–8.

MATCH. (2007) *Multidisciplinary Assessment of Technology Centre for Healthcare – The MATCH Programme*. <http://www.match.ac.uk/>. Accessed December 2007.

Maxwell, A. (2003) 'Industry angered by EC haste on implants directive', *Clinica Direct Daily*, 10 September 2003: 1. <http://www.quotientdiagnostics.co.uk/>.

May, C., Mort, M., Mair, F. and Williams, T. (2001) 'Factors affecting the adoption of tele-healthcare in the United Kingdom: The policy context and the problem of evidence', *Health Informatics Journal*, 7: 131–4.

May, C., Harrison, R., MacFarlane, A., Williams, T., Mair, F. and Wallace, P. (2003) 'Why do telemedicine systems fail to normalize as stable models of service delivery?', *Journal of Telemedicine and Telecare*, 9: S25-S26.

McAteer, H., Cosh, E., Freeman, G., Pandit, A., Wood, P. and Lilford, R. (2007) 'Cost-effectiveness analysis at the development phase of a potential health technology: examples based on tissue engineering of bladder and urethra', *Journal of Tissue Engineering and Regenerative Medicine*, 1 (5): 343–9.

McGrath, L. R., Shardlow, D. L., Ingham, E., Andrews, M., Ivory, J., Stone, M. H. and Fisher, J. (2001) 'A retrieval study of Capital hip prostheses with titanium alloy femoral stems', *Journal of Bone and Joint Surgery [Br]*; 83-B: 1195–201.

MDA. (1995) *Code of practice on enforcement*. Department of Health, London.

MDA. (1998a) *The medical devices vigilance system European commission guidelines*. Department of Health, London.

MDA. (1998b) *Guidance on the medical devices vigilance system for CE marked joint replacement implants*. London: MDA.

MDA. (2000) *One liners issue 9*. London: MDA.

MDA. (2000) *Equipped to Care: The safe use of medical devices in the 21st century*. London: MDA.

MDA. (2002) *Possibility of over infusions with IVAC 591,597, 598 and 599 Infusion Pumps*. London: MDA.

MDA. (2002a) *One liner: Infusion pumps*. London: MDA.

MDA. (2002b) *A Code of Practice for the Production of Human-derived Therapeutic Products*. London: Department of Health.

MDA (MHRA). (2003) *Infusion systems*. Device Bulletin DB2003(02). London: MDA.

Melia, J., Moss, S. and Johns, L. (2004) 'Rates of prostate-specific antigen testing in general practice in England and Wales in asymptomatic and symptomatic patients: a cross-sectional study', *BJU International*, 94: 51–6.

Melia, J. (2005) Part 1: 'The burden of prostate cancer, its natural history, information on the outcome of screening and estimates of ad hoc screening with particular reference to England and Wales', *BJU International*, 95: 4–15.

MHRA. (undated). *Conformity Assessment Procedures under the* In Vitro *Diagnostic Medical Devices Directive 98/79/EC*.< http://www.mstranslations.com/>.

MHRA. (2002) *Management and Use of IVD Point of Care Test Devices*. London: Department of Health.

MHRA. (2005) 'Over the counter testing kits', *Pharmaceutical Journal*, 273.

MHRA (2006) *Infusion device incident investigation guidelines*. London: MHRA.

MHRA. (2006) *Medical Device Alert, Baxter Colleague volumetric infusion pumps: all models*. MDA/2006/010. < http://www.mhra.gov.uk/>. Accessed August 2006.

Molina, A. H. (1999) 'Understanding the role of the technical in the build-up of sociotechnical constituencies', *Technovation*, 19 (1): 1–29.

Moran, M. (1999) *Governing the healthcare state: A comparative study of the United Kingdom, the United States and Germany*. Manchester: Manchester University Press.

Moran, M. (2001) 'The rise of the regulatory state in Britain', *Parliamentary Affairs*, 54 (1): 15–31.

Murray, D. W, Carr, A. J, Bulstrode, C. J. (1995) 'Which primary total hip replacement?', *Journal of Bone and Joint Surgery*, 77-B: 520–7.

Murray, E., Eitzmaurice, D., McCahon, D., Fuller, C. and Sandhur, H. (2004) 'Training for patients in a randomised controlled trail of self management of warfarin treatment', *British Medical Journal*, 328: 437–8.

National Audit Office (NAO). (2000) 'Hip replacements: getting it right first time', Report by the Comptroller and Auditor General. London: Stationery Office.

National Audit Office (NAO). (2003) 'Hip replacements: an update', Report by the Comptroller and Auditor General. London: Stationery Office.

National Audit Office (NAO). (2005) 'A Safer Place for Patients: Learning to improve patient safety', Report by the Comptroller and Auditor General. London: The Stationery Office.

National Patient Safety Agency. (2004a) *Safer practice notice – improving infusion device safety.* <www.npsa.nhs.uk>. Accessed November 2007.

National Patient Safety Agency. (2004b) 'Standardising and centralising infusion devices: a project to develop solutions for NHS trusts', Full evaluation report. London: NPSA.

Neary, F. (2007) 'From Cottage Industry to Multi-National Business: Manufacturing Total Hip Replacement – a Case of Convergence and Variety', Unpublished paper, University of Cambridge.

Neary, F. and Pickstone, J. (2007) 'Introduction', in L. A. Reyonolds and E. M. Tansey (eds). *Early development of total hip replacement.* Wellcome Witnesses to Twentieth Century Medicine, London: Wellcome Trust Centre for the History of Medicine, pp. xxv–xxix.

Newman, K. J. H. (1993) 'Total hip and knee replacements: A survey of 261 hospitals in England', *Journal of the Royal Society of Medicine*, 86: 527–9.

NHS CRD. (1997) *Effectiveness Matters. Screening for prostate cancer: the evidence. Information for men considering or asking for PSA tests.* York: University of York, NHS CRD.

NHS Executive. (2000). *The NHS Prostate Cancer Programme.* <http://www.doh.gov.uk/cancer/prostate.htm>. Accessed 17 May 2003.

NHS PASA. (2005) *Better patient safety through improved device manangement: infusion devices.* NHS PASA. <http://www.pasa.nhs.uk/>. Accessed 7 August 2006.

NHS PASA. (2007) *Purchasing for safety – Injectable medicines,* <http://www.pasa.nhs.uk/>. Accessed November 2007.

NHS Supply Chain. (2006). *ODEP Database.* http://www.supplychain.nhs.uk/>. Accessed 1 November 2007.

NHS Trust. (2006) *C257 – Guideline for Patient Self-Testing/Management of International Normalised Ratio (INR).* Bangor, Wales: North West Wales NHS.

NICE. (2000a) *Selection of artificial hip joints for primary total hip replacement – guidance from NICE.* <http://www.nice.org.uk/nice-web/>. National Institute for Clinical Excellence.

NICE. (2000b) *NICE issues guidance to the NHS on artificial hip joints.* London: National Institute of Clinical Excellence. [Press release].

NICE. (2000c) *Guidance on the Use of Autologous Cartilage Transplantation for Full Thickness Cartilage Defects in Knee Joints.* Technology Appraisal Guidance No. 16. NICE: London.

NICE. (2002) *Guidance on Cancer Services. Improving Outcomes in Urological Cancers. The Manual.* London: National Institute for Health & Clinical Excellence. <http://www.nice.org.uk/>. Accessed September 2007.

NICE. (2005a) *The use of autologous chondrocyte implantation for the treatment of cartilage defects in knee joints.* NICE Technology Appraisal 89, London: NICE.

NICE. (2005b) *NICE updates guidance on the use of autologous chondrocyte implantation in treating cartilage defects in knee joints,* Press Release 25 May 2005 <http://www.nice.org.uk/>.

NJR Centre – National Joint Registry. (2005) Annual Report. London: NJR <www.njrcentre.org.uk>.

NJR/NAO. National Joint Registry. (2006) Annual Report. London: NJR <www.njrcentre.org.uk>.

NJR (2007) Annual Report. London: NJR <www.njrcentre.org.uk>.

Novas, C. (2006) 'The Political Economy of Hope: Patients' Organizations, Science and Biovalue', *BioSocieties*, 1: 289–305.

Oliver, S. E., May, M. T. and Gunnell, D. (2001) 'International trends in prostate-cancer mortality in the "PSA ERA"', *International Journal of Cancer*, 92: 893–8.

Oliver, S. E., Donovan, J. L., Peters, T. J.,Frankel, S.,Hamdy, F. C. and Neal, D. E. (2003) 'Recent trends in the use of radical prostatectomy in England: the epidemiology of diffusion', *BJU International*, 91 (4): 331–6.

Oudshoorn, N. and Pinch, T. J. (eds). (2003) *How users matter: The co-construction of users and technologies*, Cambridge, MA; London: MIT Press.

Padeletti, L. (2006) 'Pacemaker selection: time for a rethinking of complex pacing systems: reply', *European Heart Journal*, 27 (9): 1127.

Pandit, H. G., Hand, C. J., Ramos, J. L., Pradhan, N. S. and Hobbs, N. J. (2000) 'Early aseptic loosening in one design (3M-Capital) of cemented total hip replacement', *Hip International*, 10 (1): 38–42.

Parliamentary Office of Science and Technology (POST). (2003) *Postnote Medical Self-test Kits.* London: POST.

Paul, J. P. (1997) 'Development of standards for orthopaedic implants', *Proceedings of the Institution of Mechanical Engineers*, Part H, 211 (1): 119–26.

Petersen, A. (1996) 'Risk and the regulated self: the discourse of health promotion as politics of uncertainty', *Australian and New Zealand Journal of Sociology*, 32 (1): 44–57.

Perrow, C. (1999) *Normal accidents: Living with high-risk technologies*. Princeton: Princeton University Press.

Pickstone, J. (2006) 'Bones in Lancashire: Towards Long-Term Contextual Analysis of Medical Technology', in C. Timmermans and J. Anderson (eds). *Devices and Designs: Medical Technologies in Historical Perspective*. Basingstoke: Palgrave Macmillan, pp. 17–36.

Pickstone, M. and Quinn, C. (2002) 'Making IV therapy safer: competence training, safety culture and technology', in Emslie et al., (eds). (2002) *Improving patient safety: Insights from American, Australian and British health care*. Based on the proceedings of a joint ECRI and Department of Health conference to introduce the National Patient Safety Agency. Welwyn Garden City: ECRI Europe.

Pinch, T. (2003) 'Giving birth to new users: how the Minimoog was sold to Rock and Roll', in Oudshoorn and Pinch (eds), pp. 247–70.

Pinch, T., Ashmore, M. and Mulkay, M. (1992) 'Technology, testing, text: Clinical budgeting in the UK National Health Service', in W. E. Bijker and J. Law (eds), *Shaping Technology/Building Society: Studies in Sociotechnical Change*. Cambridge: MIT Press.

Pirovano, D. (2007) *Eucomed position on Advanced Therapies*, Presentation at TOPRA Medical Technologies Symposium: Regulatory Affairs Challenges through to 2010. <www.topra.org>. Accessed November 2007.

Pons, J., Marti Valls, J. and Gradados, A. (1999) *Elements for the improvement of effectiveness and efficiency in hip prosthetic replacement*. Barcelona: Catalan Agency for Health Technology Assessment and Research.

Rabeharisoa,V. and Callon, M. (2002) 'The involvement of patients' associations in research', *International Social Science Journal*, 54 (171): 57–63.

Ram, M. B., Browne, N., Grocott, P. and Weir, H. (2005) *Methods to capture user perspectives in the medical device technology lifecycle: A review of the literature in health care, social science, and engineering & ergonomics*. MATCH – Multidisciplinary Assessment of Technology Centre for Health.<http://www.match.ac.uk>.

Ramlogan, R., Mina, A., Tampubolon, G. and Metcalfe, J. S. (2007) 'Networks of knowledge: The distributed nature of medical innovation', *Scientometrics*, 70 (2): 459–89.

RCS. (2001) *An investigation of the performance of the 3M capital hip system*. Royal College of Surgeons, London.

Redekop, W. K., McDonnell, J., Verboom, P., Lovas, K. and Kalo, Z. (2003) 'The Cost Effectiveness of Apligraf[(R)] Treatment of Diabetic Foot Ulcers', *Pharmacoeconomics*, 21 (16): 1171–83.

Reynolds, L. A. and Tansey, E. M. (eds). (2007) *Early development of total hip replacement*. Wellcome Witness Seminars, no. 29, London, The Wellcome Trust Centre for the History of Medicine.

Rhodes, R. A. W. (1997) *Understanding governance: policy networks, reflexivity and accountability*. Buckingham: Open University Press.

Roberts, M. (2004) 'Prostate cancer testing quandary', *BBC News Health*, 13 August 2004. <http://news.bbc.co.uk/>. Accessed August 2007.

Robertson, A. (2000) 'Embodying risk, embodying political rationality: Women's accounts of risk for breast cancer', *Health, Risk and Society*, 2 (2): 219–35.

Roche Dignostics. (2006) <www.roche-diagnostics.co.uk>. Accessed October 2006.

Rose, D. and Blume, S. (2003) 'Citizens as users of technology: An exploratory study of vaccines and vaccination', in N. Oudshoorn and T. Pinch (eds). *How Users Matter*, pp. 103–31.

Roy, N., Hossain, S., Ayeko, C., McGee, H. M., Elsworth, C. F. and Jacobs, L. G. H. (2002) '3M Capital hip arthroplasty', *Acta Orthopaedica Scandinavica*, 73 (4): 400–2.

Royal College of Nursing (RCN). (2003) 'UK Standards for intravenous therapy', London: RCN.

Runciman, W. B. (2002) 'Lessons from Austrialia', in Emslie, Knox, Pickstone (eds).

Russell, S. and Williams, R. (1988) *Opening the Black Box and Closing it Behind You: On Microsociology in the Social Analysis of Technology*, University of Edinburgh: Research Centre for Social Sciences.

Ryan, A., Wilson, S., Greenfield, S., Clifford, S., McManus, R. J. and Pattison, H. M. (2006) 'Range of self-tests available to buy in the United Kingdom: An Internet survey', *Journal of Public Health*, 28 (4): 370–4.

saferhealthcare.org. (2006) *What support services? Three patients describe their experience of using warfarin.* <http://www.saferhealthcare.org.uk/>: saferhealthcare.org.

Sarmiento, A. (2003). 'The Relationship Between Orthopaedics and Industry Must Be Reformed', *Clinical Orthopaedics and Related Research*, 412: 38–44.

Savage, P., Bates, C., Abel, P. and Waxman, J. (1997) 'British urological surgery practice: 1. Prostate cancer', *British Journal of Urology*, 79 (5): 749–54.

Sawicki, P. (2001) 'Evidence levels in recommendations for self management of oral anticoagulation', *British Medical Journal*, <http://www.bmj.com/cgi/eletters/323/7319/985#17617>, Accessed July 2007.

Sawicki, P. T. (1999) 'A structured teaching and self-management program for patients receiving oral anticoagulation – A randomized controlled trial', *JAMA-Journal of the American Medical Association*, 281: 145–50.

Scales, J. T. (1965) 'Arthroplasty of the hip using foreign materials: a history', *Proceedings of the Institution of Mechanical Engineers*, 181 (3): 63–84.

Schaeffer, C. (2007) 'Quality of life and self-monitoring: CVD prevention in practice. The role of patient organizations in CVD', *European Heart Journal* (Supplements), 9-B: B42-B44.

Schutte, E. (2003) 'Industry position on proposed directive' (representing Eucomed), Presentation at Public Hearing Quality and Safety of Human Tissue and Cells, European Parliament, Brussels, 29 January 2003. http://www.eutop.de/ct/. Accessed June 2004.

Schwartz Cowan, R. (1987) 'The consumption junction: A proposal for research strategies in the sociology of technology', in W. E. Bijker, T. P. Hughes and T. J. Pinch, (1987)(eds) *The social construction of technological systems: New directions in the sociology and history of technology*, Cambridge, MA; London: MIT Press, pp. 261–80.

Scientific Committee on Medicinal Products and Medical Devices (SCMPMD). (2001) *Opinion on the State of the Art Concerning Tissue Engineering*. <http://europa.eu.int/comm/>. Accessed 18 March 2003.

Selley, S., Donovan, J., Faulkner, A., Coast, J. and Gillatt, D. (1997) 'Diagnosis, management and screening of early localised prostate cancer', *Health Technology Assessment*, 1 (2): 1–96 (whole volume).

Shah, S. G. S. and Robinson, I. (2007) 'Benefits of and barriers to involving users in medical device technology development and evaluation', *International Journal of Technology Assessment in Health Care*, 23 (1): 131–7.

Sherriff, R., Best, L., Roderick, P. (1998) 'Population screening in the NHS: a systematic pathway from evidence to policy formulation', *Journal of Public Health Medicine*, 20 (1): 58–62.

Silverman, D. (1997). *Discourses of Counselling: HIV Counselling as Social Interaction*. London: Sage.

Silverstone, R. and Haddon, L. (1996) 'Design and the Domestication of Information and Communication technologies: Technical Change and Everyday Life', in *Communication by Design*. Oxford: Oxford University Press, pp. 44–74.

Skryabina, E. (2004) *Baxter Flo-Gard GSP syringe pump*. Bath: Bath Institute of Medical Engineering.

Smith, R. (2007) 'Malignant tales', *Guardianunlimited*, <http://commentisfree. guardian.co.uk/>. Accessed October 2007.

Souza, Mara Clécia Dantas (2007) 'Regulação sanitária de produtos para a saúde no Brasil e no Reino Unido: o caso dos equipamentos eletromédicos (Medical devices regulation in Brazil and in the United Kingdom: the electromedical equipment case)'. PhD Thesis, Federal University of Bahia, Salvador, 30 March 2007.

Stamey, T. A., Caldwell, M., Mcneal, J. E., Nolley, R., Hemenez, M. and Downs, J. (2004) 'The prostate specific antigen era in the United States is over for prostate cancer: what happened in the last 20 years?', *The Journal of Urology* 172: 1297–301.

Steffen, M., Lamping, W. and Lehto, J. (2005) 'Introduction: The Europeanization of health policies', in M. Steffen (ed.). (2005) *Health Governance in Europe: Issues, Challenges and Theories*. London: Routledge.

Stewart, J. and Williams, R. (2005) 'The Wrong Trousers? Beyond the Design Fallacy: Social Learning and the User', in H. Rohracher (ed.) (2005) *User involvement in innovation processes: Strategies and limitations from a sociotechnical perspective*, Munich: Profil-Verlag, pp. 195–221.

Styles, C. M., Evans, S. C. and Gregson, P. J. (1998) 'Development of fatigue lifetime predictive test methods for hip implants', *Biomaterials*, 19 (11–12): 1057–65.

Swan, J., Newell, S., Robertson, M., Goussevskaia, A. and Bresnen, M. (2007) 'The role of institutional differences in biomedical innovation processes: A comparison of the UK and US', *International Journal of Healthcare Technology and Management*, 8(3–4): 333–53.

Sweetnam, D. R. (1981) 'A surveillance scheme with "Recommended List" of artificial joints', *Health Trends*, 13: 43–4.

Tang, E., Lai, C. S. M., Lee, K. K. C., Wong, R. S. M., Cheng, G. and Chan, T. Y. K. (2003) 'Relationship between patients' warfarin knowledge and anticoagulation control', *Annals of Pharmacotherapy*, 37: 34–9.

Taxis, K. (2005). 'Who is responsible for the safety of infusion devices? It's high time for action!', *Quality and Safety in Health Care*, 14: 76.

Taxis, K. and Barber, N. (2003) 'Ethnographic study of incidence and severity of intravenous drug errors', *British Medical Journal*, 326: 684–7.

Thornton, H. and Dixon-Woods, M. (2002) 'Prostate specific antigen testing for prostate cancer', *British Medical Journal*, 325: 725–6.

Timmermans, S. and Berg, M. (2003a) 'The practice of medical technology', *Sociology of Health & Illness*, 25 (3): 97–114.

Timmermans, S. and Berg, M. (2003b) *The gold standard: the challenge of evidence-based medicine and standardization in health care*. Philadelphia: Temple University Press.

Tsien, C. and Fackler, J. (2004) 'Poor prognosis for existing monitors in the intensive care unit', *Critical Care Medicine*, 25 (4): 614–9.

Vahatalo, M. A., Virtamo, H. E., Viikari, J. S. and Ronnemaa, T. (2004) 'Cellular phone transferred self blood glucose monitoring: Prerequisites for positive outcome', *Practical Diabetes International*, 21 (5): 192–4.

van der Meulen, J. (2005) *Current practice in the assessment of joint prostheses: Strength and weaknesses in existing performance data*, <www.bitecic.com/events/Meulen1%20-%20London15Sept2005_1.pdf>. Accessed July 2007.

van Merkerk, R. O. and van Lente, H. (2005) 'Tracing emerging irreversibilities in emerging technologies: The case of nanotubes', *Technological Forecasting and Social Change*, 72, 9: 1094–111.

van Merkerk, R. O. and Robinson, D. K. R. (2006) 'Characterizing the Emergence of a Technological Field: Expectations, Agendas and Networks in Lab-on-a-chip Technologies', *Technology Analysis & Strategic Management*, 18 (3/4): 411–28.

van Merode, G. G., Adang, E. M. M. and Paulus, A. T. G. (2002) 'Innovation in the medical device industry', *International Journal of Healthcare Technology and Management*, 4 (5): 333–49.

Vincent, C. H., Taylor-Adams, S. and Stanhope, N. (1998) 'Framework For Analysing Risk and Safety In Clinical Medicine', *British Medical Journal*, 316: 1154–7.

Vogel, D. (2001) 'The new politics of risk regulation in Europe', CARR Discussion paper 3, London School of Economics.

Waldby, C. (2002a) 'Stem Cells, Tissue Cultures and the Production of Biovalue', *Health: An Interdisciplinary Journal for the Social Study of Health, Illness and Medicine*, 6 (3): 305–23.

Waldby, C. (2002b) 'Biomedicine, Tissue Transfer and Intercorporeality', *Feminist Theory*, 3 (3): 239–54.

Wang, M. C., Valenzuela, L. A., Murphy, G. P. and Chu, T. M. (1979) 'Purification of a Human-Prostate Specific Antigen', *Investigative Urology*, 17: 159–63.

Wanless, D. (2002) 'Securing Our Future Health: Taking a Long-Term View'. <http://www.hm-treasury.gov.uk/>. Accessed July 2007.

Watson, E., Jenkins, L., Bukach, C. and Austoker, J. (2002) 'The PSA test and prostate cancer: information for primary care', NHS Cancer Screening Programmes, Sheffield. <http://www.cancerscreening.nhs.uk/prostate/>. Accessed July 2007.

Waugh, W. (1990) *John Charnley: The man and the hip*. Berlin: Springer-Verlag.

Wearne, P. and Jones, J. (1993) 'Shooting at the Hip – Shoddy material and inept surgeons mean that up to 30% of hip replacements have to be redone', *Guardian*, 23 February 1993.

Webster, A. (1994) 'University-corporate ties and the construction of research agendas', *Sociology*, 28 (1): 123–42.

Webster, A. (2002) 'Innovative health technologies and the social: redefining health, medicine and the body'. *Current Sociology*, 50: 443–58.

Webster, A. (2004a) 'Health technology assessment: A sociological commentary on reflexive innovation', *International Journal of Technology Assessment in Health Care*, 20 (1): 1–6.

Webster, A. (2004b) 'State of the Art: Risk, science and policy – researching the social management of uncertainty', *Policy Studies*, 25: 5–18.

Webster, A. (2007) *Health, Technology and Society: A sociological critique*. Basingstoke: Palgrave Macmillan.

Weller, D., May, F., Rowett, D., Esterman, A., Pinnock, C., Nicholson, S., Doust, J. and Silagy, C. (2003) 'Promoting better use of the PSA test in general practice: RCT of educational strategies based on outreach visit and mailout', *Family Practice*, 20 (6): 655–61.

Wennberg, J. E., Freeman, J. L. and Culp, W. J. (1987) 'Are hospital services rationed in New Haven or over-utilised in Boston?', *Lancet*, 23 May, 1 (8543): 1185–9.

Wennberg, J. and Gittelsohn, A. (1982) 'Variations in medical care among small areas', *Scientific American*, 246: 100–12.

Wilson, S., Greenfield, S., Pattison, H. M., Ryan, A., McManus, R. M., Fitzmaurice, D., Marriott, J., Chapman, C. and Clifford, S. (2006) 'Prevalence of the use of cancer related self-tests by members of the public: a community survey', *BMC Cancer*, 6: 215.

Winner, L. (1985) 'Do artifacts have politics?' in D. A. MacKenzie and J. Wajcman (eds), *The social shaping of technology: How the refrigerator got its hum*. Milton Keynes: Open University Press.

Winslow, M., Clark, D., Seymour, J., Noble, W., ten Have, H., Meldrum, M. and Paz, S. (2003) 'Changing technologies of cancer pain relief: themes from the twentieth century', *Progress in Palliative Care*, 11 (5): 1–5.

Wirtz, V., Taxis, K. and Narber, N. D. (2003) 'An observational study of IV medication errors in the UK and Germany', *Pharm World Sci*, 25: 104–11.

WMHTAC. (2007) 'What is the cost effectiveness of self-monitoring and self-management of anticoagulation treatment compared with clinic based monitoring?' <http://www.hta.nhsweb.nhs.uk/>. Accessed June 2007.

Woolf, S. H. and Henshall, C. (2000) 'Health technology assessment in the United Kingdom', *International Journal of Technology Assessment in Health Care*, 16: 591–625.

Woolgar, S. (1991) 'Configuring the user: The case of usability trials', in J. Law, (ed.). *A sociology of monsters*, London: Routledge, pp. 58–99.

World Health Organization. (2003) 'Medical device regulations: Global overview and guiding principles'. Geneva: World Health Organization.

Index